REGAN
ARCHIBALD

REGAN ARCHIBALD

THE PEPTIDE BLUEPRINT

Achieving Optimal Health and Performance at Any Age

REGAN ARCHIBALD, Lac, FMP

Library of Congress Control Number:

ISBN: 9-798-39729013-5

Printed in the United States of America.

CONTENTS

YOUR HEALTH CAN'T WAIT   1

A CAUTIONARY TALE (OR THREE)   7
"I Can't Tie My Shoes"   7
The Signs You Can't Ignore   10
It's Almost Never Too Late   13

FROM FARM TO FITNESS   19

WHAT IS ACCELERATE WELLNESS?   25
The Importance of Communication   26
What's In Store for You   29
What's Different About Accelerate Wellness?   31

THE "MAGIC" OF PEPTIDES   37
What Is a Peptide?   38
Where Did They Come From?   40
Cleaning Up the Body's Processes   41
Why Peptides?   43
The Bottom Line   44
Making the Most of Peptides   46
What Are They Good for?   46
Okay, Which Ones Do I Need?   48

DEEP DIVE: RESET   51

DEEP DIVE: RECHARGE   67

DEEP DIVE: RESTORE   83

PUTTING IT ALL TOGETHER   101

What Happens When You Work With Us   103

Testing, Testing   104

Your Personal Accelerate Wellness Team   106

The Secret to Your Success   108

WHAT'S NEXT?   111

Health Optimization and Age Reversal   112

Peak State Experience   113

Always Another Step   115

APPENDIX A: PEPTIDES   117

HPA Stress Reset   117

Lean Muscle + Endurance   119

Immune Reset   121

Your Best Weight   123

Gut Recharge   125

Inner Genius   127

Energy + Mito Restore   129

Pain + Regeneration   131

Cognitive Reclamation   133

Sexual Rejuvenation   135

APPENDIX B: FITNESS 50 BENCHMARKS   138

WORK WITH REGAN AND THE EAST WEST

HEALTH TEAM   142

ABOUT REGAN ARCHIBALD   143

ENDNOTES   145

YOUR HEALTH CAN'T WAIT

Most people have no idea what great health feels like. We have no idea that the normal state of life is not morning aches and pains, afternoon fog, and a restless night of tossing and turning and interrupted sleep — if we manage to get to sleep at all.

Instead, the average American self-medicates with over-the-counter pain relievers to banish stiffness, caffeine to jumpstart the ol' energy and fight the post-lunch slump, a glass of wine or a beer or three to unwind, and sleep aids at bedtime to (hopefully) knock us out so we can finally get some rest and counteract the junk we've been putting into our bodies over the last 12 to 14 hours of the day. Then we wake up groggy the next morning and start the routine all over again. That's just life, right?

Wrong.

The reason I write books, record podcasts, and consult with patients is that a lot of people are unhealthy, and I don't want you to be one of them.

As the founder of East West Health, I focus on age reversal — allowing you to become unreasonably healthy in the shortest amount of time, without sacrificing the parts of life you enjoy the most.

The truth is that we were created to live a long, vibrant life, one free of the pain, discomfort, and disease that we've begun to take as a normal and natural part of living. Yes, aging does bring with it some changes to our bodies and minds, but much of what we consider unavoidable is actually preventable or delayable, if we take the right steps while there's still time.

I'm a firm believer that we can all do better than our current "average," and the time to do something about it is **now**. Your time is the most valuable resource you have. I want to take the guesswork out of staying healthy, so I've used my missteps and false starts as a way to save you time so you can make your next decade of life — however old you are now — your *best* decade.

Health is an investment. We often don't realize its importance until something threatens it. But one phone call from the doctor, one scary test result, and we suddenly realize how precious our health is — and how much we've taken it for granted. Then we wish we'd paid attention to what our bodies had been telling us when we still could do something about it.

Unfortunately, many of us put our most valuable resource in a very risky position. We've been fooling ourselves into thinking that we are healthier than we really are, and that the declines and issues we've been experiencing are nothing more than what's to be expected.

The challenge with this perspective is that when we adopt a hands-off, fatalistic approach to our health, we are putting *everything* on the line. Once you've had a heart attack or cancer or have been diagnosed with diabetes, you can't take back the years spent living a sub-optimal lifestyle, or the time you could have been making small changes that could have had a large impact on the quality of your life. In other words, you don't have to make huge adjustments to reap major rewards.

In fact, data gathered in 2017 by the Health and Retirement Study[1] found that people who are 50 and older who were normal weight, had never smoked, and had kept their alcohol consumption moderate lived on average seven years longer than those who were overweight, smokers, and heavy drinkers.

The research doesn't stop there. A 2012 metaanalysis of 15 international studies,[2] which included more than 500,000 participants, found that over half of premature deaths were due to unhealthy lifestyle factors such as poor diet, inactivity, obesity, excessive alcohol intake, and smoking.

In other words, just by not smoking, drinking moderately, and adopting a more nutritious diet, you can add years to your life — and that's without any other interventions, protocols, or habit changes. When you layer on some of the exciting scientific discoveries in fields like peptides, the impact can be even greater!

The biggest surprise for you may be that it doesn't take much time for your body to begin to recover — you can feel a difference in just a few weeks! Our natural state is wellness, not disease. When we give ourselves the materials we need to operate at our natural, optimal state, we can see changes quickly, even after years of poor nutrition, overindulgence, and a sedentary lifestyle.

East West Health's Three Guiding Principles

- **Your Next Decade, Your Best Decade** – We love generating life-long relationships with everyone that we work with.
- **No Death by Neglect, No Surprises** – Get the right tests, and the right treatments, ahead of time.
- **Health Improves Everything** – Be unreasonably healthy, at any age, even if everyone around you isn't.

My purpose in writing this book is to present a new way of living to you, one that allows you to live a vibrant life as long as you wish. I want to challenge the common perceptions that are keeping many Americans stuck, sick, and sore in the area of health, even while our standard of living has risen in so many other areas. I want to open up new possibilities to you, introducing you to the idea that getting older does not have to mean giving up an active, healthy lifestyle (in fact, if you follow the suggestions in this book, you may find yourself feeling better than you ever have before — even when you were in your "prime!").

We're going to cover a lot of ground. We'll discuss how our current medical and "health"care system is failing Americans. I do this not in order to scare you, but so we can get a good grip on the challenges that face us. Then we'll talk about a new approach to health, one that enhances your body's ability to heal and protect itself. In the upcoming chapters, you will learn about some of these exciting discoveries in optimizing health and longevity, such as brand-new peptide therapies like Epitalon. Next, I'll introduce you to my three-phase Accelerate Wellness program for Resetting, Recharging, and Restoring your health, by turning on genes that express health and vitality — reversing years (and sometimes decades) of neglect in just seven months. Finally, you'll see what you need to do to immediately begin your personal transformation from "average" to a life filled with energy, health, and vibrancy.

We live in one of the richest nations in the world, with unlimited opportunity — and that includes the opportunity to live a long, healthy life. While the path most of us are on is headed toward a decline as we age, you don't have to continue to follow that downward-sloping line. With the right information and the right plan, you can completely change the course of your years. I'll show you how.

Regan Archibald, Lac, FMP
Founder, East West Health

P.S. If you're a business owner or executive, in an entrepreneurial household, or you want to reverse your aging process and get better answers so that you can feel, look, and perform your best, see our special offer in the back of this book for more information.

Your Turn

Take a moment and write down what has been lost in not having started to work on your health sooner. This is so important, so do not skip this! Ask yourself honestly, "What have I robbed myself of in the past by not handling my concerns about my health in the moment?"

_____

_____

_____

_____

Now, set your goal(s) for this challenge. What would you like to experience or realize by the end of the next seven months?

_____

_____

_____

_____

Next, use the space below to make some notes today so that you have trackable measurements of where you are now. Step one of any goal is to know your current baseline objectively. Tracking and seeing your progress from beginning to end is a powerful accountability tool and reward mechanism in and of itself. Remember, no shame, judgment, or guilt.

_____

_____

_____

_____

NOTE: Getting blood work read by a functional medicine practitioner is the best place to start. The team at East West Health would be honored to help you. See our special offer in the back of this book for more information!

CHAPTER 1

A CAUTIONARY TALE (OR THREE)

A lot of entrepreneurs and their partners or spouses — high-performers who have pushed themselves for decades — shut out everything their body is telling them to prioritize their business or care for their family, thinking that they'll have time "later" to deal with the discomfort, pain, weight gain, or other issues that have been creeping up on them. These are some of their stories, with names and identifying characteristics changed for patient confidentiality.

"I CAN'T TIE MY SHOES"

Bill is a typical founder/entrepreneur. After working diligently to build his architecture firm, at age 68 he was ready to sell and enjoy the fruits of his labor. Unfortunately, he'd ignored his health for decades, and his body wasn't cooperating. When Bill was ready to make a healthy change, he said, "Look, I've got to golf again. My belly's in the way, I can't tie my shoes, and my energy has tanked."

His complaints went beyond not being able to tie his

shoes, though. He had osteoarthritic knees. He'd lost stamina and sex drive and was experiencing various aches and pains. After running the right labs and digging a little deeper, it was discovered that Bill also had some gut issues that he hadn't disclosed; something that's very common. To deal with his discomfort, he was on about six different medications, both over-the-counter and prescription. He took Pepto Bismol to address the intestinal issues, omeprazole for acid reflux, and statin for high cholesterol. He took medicine for high blood pressure to keep his cardiovascular system functioning. But these were all just bandaids to cover the real issues. His guts were wrecked. His nervous system was in overdrive. And his hemoglobin A1C, which is a measure of the sugar in the blood, was in the pre-diabetic range.

The Accelerate Wellness protocol includes both lifestyle changes and supplementation by way of peptides and other regenerative health treatments. After implementing the protocol, Bill slowly started losing weight. He also took a peptide called Selank, a nasal spray, like a natural benzodiazepine for GABA receptors in the brain. After taking a little oxytocin, Bill suddenly felt more like himself again. Then he took Epitalon, so his sleep patterns were better, energy started returning, and his stress was abating. It changed his whole outlook on life.

After experiencing some initial healthy effects, Bill was anxious to get started on what he saw as the "real" problem — his weight. It was explained to him that there was much-needed upstream work to address first, including lowering his stress and making sure he was sleeping better to create a strong foundation for future improvements.

It wasn't until about the second month that he began to see the weight coming off. About 90 days after he started, Bill pulled up his shirt, and said, "Look at my belly!" The Santa Claus belly was gone.

Bill's biggest reward happened when he and his wife sat down to review his new blood labs. "You've done great with keeping up on your side of the deal," his health advisor told him. It's not always easy to eat the right foods, keep regular appointments with your health advisor, and follow the protocols for the Accelerate Wellness program as you develop new habits, but Bill had gone all-in. Now, his new blood labs were his report card. Would his labs support the progress he felt he'd been making?

It wasn't long after reviewing his lab results that this tough businessman was getting a bit emotional. He pointed to the green thumbs up next to his A1C, glucose, ALT, anion gap, and several other markers. "That green thumb represents progress, Bill," he was told. "The best part is, those are the changes that will last because you've gained new habits and skills that support your health. Now they are yours for the rest of your life."

In addition to the internal changes that his labs demonstrated, Bill had other improvements as well. Bill's knees went from being swollen and painful by the end of each day to having no pain at all (even after 18 holes of golf!). He achieved his weight loss goal of 30 pounds and is now in the Optimized program, building more muscle mass. He says he feels 30 years younger because of the improvements in his energy levels and sleep. He's off all of his medications now, and both he and his primary care physician are thrilled at the momentum that Bill has created in his health in a short amount of time.

In his initial meeting, Bill had expressed concerns about losing his memory and mental edge. As part of his program, peptide stacks were used to address this concern, and within a few days he was able to regain some of the focus that he felt was missing. He enjoys reading again and has even regained his confidence in keeping up his end while having more intellectual, intense conversations. He's enjoying using his architecture skills again and is even doing some side projects, and he feels like his mental and physical performance are steadily improving. He truly exhibits the goal of making his next decade, his best decade.

THE SIGNS YOU CAN'T IGNORE

In Bill's case, his desire to stay active was the impetus that brought him to seek out some help. Unfortunately, in other cases, people only seek help because of an acute issue or adverse health event they simply can't ignore. And those never, ever come at a convenient time.

This was the situation with Nancy. She was "the family boss." Now in her late 60s, she was the keeper of the house and home, and her support with the family enabled her husband to spend the majority of his energy building his business. It was an arrangement that worked well for them as Nancy raised six children, ran the household, and always kept the family on track.

Like many caregivers, she put her health on the backburner… until she was forced to pay attention.

Nancy sought help because she'd been experiencing some concerning health symptoms, including shortness of breath, overall lethargy, and a host of other seemingly unrelated concerns. After seeing a variety of doctors, Nancy ended up sitting in a cardiologist's office being told she needed a pacemaker or she faced a future fatal heart attack. Talk about a wake-up call. Heart disease ran in both sides of her family, and her father had died from a heart attack when he was only 58. Here she was, turning the corner to 70, faced with the same outlook.

Fortunately, she heard about the Accelerate Wellness program through a friend and made an appointment. She reported that her energy was dropping over the course of the day, and she was struggling to keep up with her kids and grandkids. She had just turned 70 and stated, "I feel older than dirt and gain weight just by looking at food, but there's no way I can risk having a heart attack." Even though she was going to the gym several times a week, she couldn't lose the unwanted weight that had crept on over the years. Her hair was thinning, and after her cardiologist's report, she knew she needed to change something.

A full blood panel was conducted and revealed some other unwelcome surprises. Not only was Nancy on the verge of heart failure, but she also had undiagnosed diabetes (side note: the CDC estimates that some 7 million Americans — 2.8 percent of the 18-and-over population in the U.S. — have undiagnosed diabetes. That's in addition to the 35 million who have been diagnosed![3]).

In addition to her diabetes, she was about 50 pounds overweight. Her knees, shoulders, and hips were also in almost constant pain and kept her from many activities. Add on to that the wear and tear from birthing a half-dozen children… there was a lot going on in her body.

Nancy started following the Accelerate Wellness protocol and it wasn't long before her biggest obstacle showed up: Time. It was difficult for her to remember to inject her peptides at the right time, and finding time to prepare healthy meals was also proving to be very challenging. Andie and Jeni, Nancy's health advisors, created automated text reminders for Nancy and also taught her meal prep secrets so she could get delicious meals on the table in just a few minutes.

Trysten, her fitness advisor, helped her increase strength and flexibility. After just a few weeks, she felt significantly better, with fewer food cravings, better digestion, and fewer aches and pains. She had also begun to release some of the unwanted weight that had previously been so stubborn and resistant to exercise. The real test, though, would be the results of her labs. To ensure that Nancy was moving in the right direction, she was advised, "Go see your cardiologist and show him where you are. If this isn't working, we'll need to figure out something else."

The cardiologist ran new labs and could hardly believe it. He took the time to drop a note and say, "Hey, I don't know what Nancy has been doing, but she no longer has cardiovascular disease and doesn't need a pacemaker." Needless to say, everyone was ecstatic.

The changes have continued. She's lost about 40 lbs to date, and more importantly, she feels better, has her vitality back, and is enjoying her life and her family.

IT'S ALMOST NEVER TOO LATE

The Accelerate Wellness program welcomes working with people at all stages in their lives and health journeys, from 9 to 103 (seriously!). Some are interested in fine-tuning and creating optimal health, while others are coming back from significant adverse health issues. This chapter features two stories of people who had more severe issues and who were in their 60s and early 70s. These inspiring testimonies greatly illustrate how it is never too late to make improvements in your lifestyle.

A lot of people say, "It's too late. I'm too old. I'm too fat. I'm too far gone. My time has come and passed. This is just the way it's going to be."

Many times that is not true. Sometimes, however, there are people who cannot be helped. They describe their symptoms, labs are run, and there is no clear pattern to indicate a path of treatment. In that case, it is explained to them that there is not a confident plan of action to implement. But the majority of people can be helped — even those who are at the extreme end of issues, people who are 50, 60, 70 lbs overweight or more, people with a host of seemingly unrelated symptoms, people who have pushed themselves for decades, people who are swallowing handfuls of medication every morning. So while not everyone can be helped, there is a very good chance you can be helped.

When people say that they believe they're "too far gone," Fred's story is a great example to consider. Fred is an accomplished trial lawyer in his early 60s who runs a big law firm. You can imagine the stress levels have been imposed on him.

When Fred first came in, he was severely swollen. It was absolutely the first thing you saw about him — you could just tell he wasn't healthy. There was a high concern that he could stroke out at any moment, and he was pointedly asked, "Have you ever had a stroke?"

Fred's energy was intense. He had a huge ego and was running hot. He said, "I don't want any doctor to tell me what to eat and what not to eat." His ego kept him from asking for and accepting help.

To help him, some barriers definitely needed to be broken down and trust established, which was achieved by giving him the straight facts. "You are not going to be told what to do, but by looking at your labs, you're a stroke waiting to happen. You're actually a liability for any health professional right now."

He had an important choice to make. Right in that moment, he could make some changes, but if he waited too long, that choice would be taken from him. There absolutely is a point where it's too late. An estimated 40-50 percent of heart attacks end in death, and many have no warning.[4] Fred was told, "You can be helped now, but it would have been ideal to have seen you 20 years ago. Imagine how much better your career would have been."

Fred grew up in Idaho where he had learned the value of hard work very early on. He admitted that while he had learned to stand up for himself and be a "tough guy," what worked in the courtroom didn't always work in his personal life. He had been married three times and didn't have a great relationship with his four kids, though it was clear he loved them and lit up at the mention of his grandkids. It was clear that Fred was ready for a transformation spiritually as much as he was physically.

After the kind of future that he was facing was explained to him, Fred was all in. He even said, "I'm ready to give this a try, and I actually have some hope. That hasn't happened in a long time."

It didn't take long for Fred to start feeling better. In the first 60-day phase, Reset, he started sleeping better, noticed a drop in his blood pressure, and even felt like he had more room to breathe, presumably from a drop in stress. By the end of this phase, Fred had already lost 15 pounds and felt ten years younger.

His next 60-day phase, Recharge, included a gut protocol. By the end of his liver and gut cleanse, Fred's face was noticeably thinner. The puffiness in his face was directly correlated to poor detoxification, which backs up fluid in the lymphatic system and can increase facial edema.

By Phase 3: Restore, Fred felt like he had the essentials down and he was ready to start focusing on muscle building, endurance, and coordination. When his fitness advisor took him through the benchmarks at the beginning of the program, Fred didn't even make it to the lowest level, but he didn't let that discourage him. He kept pushing himself beyond his comfort zone and made improvements.

After the full seven months, a fresh set of blood labs were ordered, and the contrast was startling. The results proved that he had indeed made lasting changes. Fred graduated into our Age Reversal program and is doing better than ever.

Fred was recently asked what has been the most impactful takeaway from this experience, and he said, "I just can't believe how long I waited to do something about my health. I never thought a grumpy old man with nothing to live for could make a turnaround like I have. I'm not where I want to be all the way yet, but I love the progress that I am making and so does my family."

This story is shared with you, again, not to scare you, but to paint a picture for you. You obviously can wait to deal with your health for another ten, twenty, or thirty years until your kids are grown and you're ready to sell your business. Hopefully, there will still be plenty of time to fix whatever's gone off the rails. But like with Fred, what are you sacrificing by waiting? Think about the energy, excitement, and vibrancy you're giving up now, betting that you'll have time at some unknown point in the future to deal with that achy back, those extra pounds, that high blood pressure. But what if there isn't time? What if you're one of those unlucky ones who roll the dice on your health and lose?

There's an old Chinese adage that says the best time to plant a tree was 20 years ago. The second best time is now. Consider this a personal call to act while you still have time to enjoy your life to the fullest.

Your Turn

Of the three stories shared in this chapter, which one (if any) do you most identify with, and why?

_____

_____

_____

_____

_____

_____

_____

_____

_____

_____

What objections come up in your mind as you think about making changes to your health?

- Too old

- Too late

- Too out of shape

- It will take too much work

- Additional objections:

_____

_____

_____

_____

_____

_____

_____

CHAPTER 2

FROM FARM TO FITNESS

I grew up on a farm in Idaho. As you can imagine, it was hard work, cold winters, and did I mention hard work? I actually really enjoyed it, even the hard work. Well, most of the time. One of the ways I got out of farm work was by taking part in school sports, so it wasn't long before I was on the football team and the basketball team. Between my chores and my sports, I was always concerned with physical fitness and having vitality.

When I was 13, my dad gave me a book called *The Inner Athlete* by Dan Millman, an Olympic athlete. That book changed my life. While I'd become very familiar with my physical body, I had never thought about the power of my mind. Suddenly, I was learning about visualization and how you could deploy your mind to help heal your body.

Because my schedule was pretty packed, I had a policy for myself that I didn't want any homework left after school. So during class, I'd try to memorize everything I could as quickly as possible. As soon as the bell rang, I'd do my assignments and then turn them in. I was able to make it through most of school with no homework.

Because of my interest in health and fitness, I started exploring natural medicine. I bought supplements and studied books about supplements and natural healing. I was completely fascinated. Like most people who fall in love with a topic, I couldn't keep my discoveries to myself — sometimes with, ahem, interesting results!

One time, I was reading about the cardiovascular and endurance benefits of vitamin C, so I decided my whole basketball team should take it — in massive doses. We were coming up against the number-one team in our state, and we needed an edge.

Unfortunately, my mistake became all too clear in the first quarter of the game when everybody had to run off the court because it turns out 8 grams of vitamin C can give you diarrhea pretty quickly! We didn't win that game, but it did give me a new respect for the power of natural medicine.

My interest in medicine and health has a family component. My amazing uncle, Lester J. Peterson, was a doctor. I decided I wanted to be like him when I grew up, so I studied pre-med in college. Around the same time, I got really sick. My hair was falling out. I was falling asleep in class. I was getting kind of pudgy, and none of it made any sense. I went to a bunch of different doctors, and they would look at my blood labs, say, "Everything is normal," and send me on my way. But I knew something wasn't right.

It was through my own desperation and desire for answers that I went to a naturopathic doctor who was also an acupuncturist. He was able to run the right labs, and I found out I had an autoimmune disease that was affecting my thyroid. Through naturopathic treatments, I was able to address this condition and get my health back.

What struck me is, here I was, taking all these classes in chemistry, physiology, pharmaceuticals. I went to "traditional" doctors, and none of it was able to help me. I started thinking about health in a different way, one focused on helping the body heal itself. I was doing coursework on my own body, treating my body as my laboratory.

That's when I decided that rather than pursuing the path of an MD and going to the University of Utah conventional medical school to learn allopathic medicine, I wanted to study integrated medicine and functional medicine. I ended up going to a Chinese medical school that was also connected to the North Hawaii Community Hospital. As a result of that connection, we were able to do a lot of collaboration with the hospital, learning both eastern and western medicine.

I started East West Health in 2004, and I've always incorporated both allopathic and integrated components to my practice. Over my entire career, I've always wanted to be the bridge between the western sciences and innovations. I've done over a decade of deep research in clinical studies with stem cell therapy and regenerative medicine. I combine the best of both approaches, blending integrated, functional medicine in my practice with ancient techniques. At East West, we create shortcuts by combining the medicine model with my knowledge of eastern medicine and more functional integrative medicine. For instance, we use a lot of acupuncture and Chinese herbs, but we also rely on testing. There are a lot of people in natural medicine who are not getting any results with their patients, and they can't really figure out why. I think it's because of the lack of integration. There's absolutely a place for natural medicine, but you need studies to back it up. That's why with every patient, we run blood work, we run stool tests and metabolomics, and we're looking at the environmental toxins and removing those interferences and building up deficiencies. But you can't do that confidently if you don't have a science-backed test to influence your decisions.

The bottom line is, at East West Health, the body is observed and engaged in a totally different manner than how traditional western medicine works so that people can receive personalized attention and get healthier faster.

And it works. East West Health is one of the fastest-growing virtual functional medicine clinics and one of the largest peptide clinics in the country with an unlimited growth trajectory, helping people outside the United States, in places like Canada and Italy, and as far as Pakistan. East West Health is committed to raising the bar by continuing to be very obsessive, interested, and aware of what's going on medically from a scientific perspective. Over 1500 doctors in 17 different medical curriculums are currently trained in the Accelerate Wellness program.

As a dedicated health professional, I research and study, and I also continue to experiment on myself. Every year I do different experiments. One year I wanted to test the efficacy of extreme cold, so I committed to doing 365 days of ice baths, and every day I took at least one ice bath. (By the way, it's phenomenal! I still do a lot of cold exposure, and you'll be challenged to do so in Phase 2 of the Accelerate Wellness program). I've done years where I've exercised twice a day. I do these different experiments because I believe that if you can put your body in a place where it enjoys doing physical activities and you don't stop doing those activities as you age, you will never lose your balance, never lose coordination, never lose agility, never lose strength, never lose power. Starting strong and continuing to challenge yourself is the best bet for living a super long, healthy life.

It's through this combination of eastern and western medicine, and my continued research and experimentation, that the Accelerate Wellness program was born. The goal is to have the **next decade be your best decade, no matter what age you are now.** If you're 80, allow yourself to get from 80 to 90 with your best health ever. In the next chapter, you'll learn about a much more detailed view of the Accelerate Wellness program and how it can work for you.

Your Turn

I "discovered" the power of the mind through a book that was gifted to me. It's my hope that this book you're now holding will help you discover the power of your body to heal itself. Have you experienced a "mind over body" incident (maybe in childbirth, or dealing with pain or discomfort)? Describe.

_____

_____

_____

_____

_____

_____

_____

_____

_____

What about the combination of eastern and western medicine intrigues or appeals to you?

_____

_____

_____

_____

_____

_____

_____

_____

_____

_____

CHAPTER 3

WHAT IS ACCELERATE WELLNESS?

It's not unusual for high-performing individuals to be excelling at work and in their relationships — but fail in the area of personal health. Unfortunately, as discussed in previous chapters, you can "borrow" from your health account for only so long before it catches up with you (and that never, ever happens at a "convenient" time!). The beautiful thing is, when you start making your health a priority, you will see the effects in every area of your life. Your relationships will get stronger. You'll perform better at work. And you'll have more confidence and energy to tackle any obstacle or goal in front of you. No more brain fog, afternoon slumps, or "hangry" moments... You'll be at the top of your game in every area of your life.

One of the biggest concerns with busy people when they think about adopting a new health program is, obviously, time. Sorting through all the various conflicting reports on health and fitness, fat loss, diet, exercise, integrative therapies and more can be overwhelming for anyone with a science degree, let alone someone who's trying to run a business or run a home. Most people simply don't have enough hours in the day already, without spending hours a day at the gym or preparing complicated recipes with hard-to-find ingredients.

Not only that, but people at the top of their game in business typically want the best results, fast. You want to know you're getting the latest and greatest, and that you're going to get the results you desire, in the most direct means possible.

That's why the Accelerate Wellness program, a systematic way of helping you achieve your biggest health goals, was developed. Experts in health and fitness have done the heavy lifting for you, designing an effective, simple program that will deliver results. In just seven months — three phases of 60 days each, plus a month for fine-tuning and adjustments — you'll see huge results in your energy level, body composition, bloodwork, and more. This is possible because of the belief in essentialism: the commitment to focus on what matters most — the essentials — to achieve the goals you want.

THE IMPORTANCE OF COMMUNICATION

Optimal health is not an accident. It occurs when everything is working as it should, at the most minute levels of your body, particularly in cell-to-cell communication. If this communication is interrupted in any way — because of interferences, inflammation, or toxins — cells cannot coordinate and adjust their functions. When this disruption occurs, your mitochondria (the energy motor of the cell), steps in and activates an immune response. This mitochondrial response is called "cell danger response," or CDR. When your CDR is active, your body will decrease needed hormone production and increase disease patterns and reduce ATP or cellular energy. In other words, you'll feel worn-out and tired, and you'll be more susceptible to disease.

To address the importance of cell-to-cell communication in your overall health, the Accelerate Wellness program will transform every system in your body, remove interferences and biotoxins, and turn on effective cell-to-cell communication.

The Accelerate Wellness program is organized around:

- **Removing interferences** — anything that's getting in the way of optimal health

- **Removing inflammation** — an immune response from exposure to oxidative stress

- **Removing toxins** — getting rid of chemicals that are bad for your health

- **Building up deficiencies** — identifying and addressing shortage of needed substances needed by your body to operate optimally

During the entire seven months, you will be mentored and supported to perform three core activities:

1. ANALYZE: Pinpointing barriers to healing and interferences, and finding opportunities for improvements.

2. OPTIMIZE: Detoxing pathways and prioritizing ideal nutrition, fitness, brain performance, and gut health.

3. TRANSFORM: Creating healthy lifestyle and habits, offering accountability, and monitoring progress.

If you're looking to change your life through better health — and you want to see and feel results fast — the Accelerate Wellness program is for you. To date, over 5,000 people have successfully experienced the incredible transformation to optimal wellness, using the Reset • Recharge • Restore approach to health over the last decade. Here's what the program looks like:

Phase 1: Reset

The first phase is called Reset because the goal is to return your body to its natural state. Multiple parameters of your health are looked at to reset your mind and body so that you can start maximizing your overall health as it detoxifies and heals. The focus in this 60-day phase is on HPA, detoxification, and energy.

Phase 2: Recharge

The next phase is Recharge, which focuses on DNA, gut health, and mitochondria to ensure that you're able to regain the physical stamina that you need to stay energized all day. In order to recharge the body, correcting the bacteria balance in the gut is key. Additionally, the Recharge phase is when you'll notice the biggest change in digestion. This phase often results in the disappearance of chronic bloating, indigestion, and gas completely. This is the phase when most people notice their clothes fitting differently because of the change in their body composition.

Phase 3: Restore

The final phase of the Accelerate Wellness program is Restore, where you'll focus on metabolic flexibility and age reversal, so you can cement your progress for continuing health in the years to come.

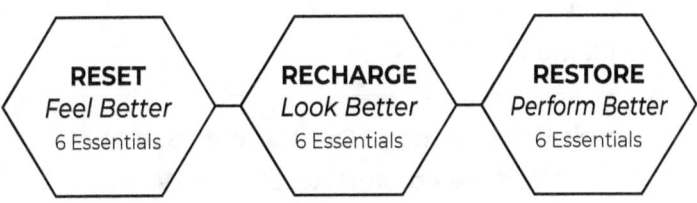

Greater detail on each of these phases is provided in the upcoming chapters. Each phase is organized into six core essentials, designed to create momentum right out of the gate and to ensure you're never guessing about what to focus on or do on a daily basis.

WHAT'S IN STORE FOR YOU

People who have taken part in the Accelerate Wellness Program have been astounded at how quickly they've seen — and more importantly, *felt* — results. Often within a matter of a week or two, you'll notice changes in your energy level. If you've been in pain or had ongoing discomfort, you'll sense that your body is healing.

Here are just a handful of the positive results you might experience:

- Reversal of disease
- Mitigation of pain and discomfort
- Weight loss
- Increased mobility and flexibility
- Greater confidence
- Better sleep
- Renewed energy
- And more!

Here's What Some of Our Patients Say About East West Health and Accelerate Wellness

"Everything is great - my relationship with my wife, no aches or pains, my flexibility is up, my weight is down. The support has been integral to making this happen! I am now teaching my children what I have learned. I am enjoying my life."

D.P., 54-year-old male

"I am so pleased with the results of my Accelerated Wellness program at East West Health. It has improved my health and relieved the pain in both of my knees. I had horrible pain in my right knee and that has improved so much - I just have small twinges now. My left knee is almost pain free. I feel very optimistic that I will progress to NO pain in time."

Vicki C., 77-year-old female

"From the moment I stepped through the door at East West Health, I was met with genuine, professional, knowledgeable and concerned people. Every aspect of the process was explained and performed perfectly. In short, I could not be happier with my decision and I am confident that because of their work my life has been changed dramatically for the better! Not only have I lost 30 pounds by following their Accelerate Wellness program, but I look 10 years younger and feel the best I have in decades. My business has never been more successful and because of my health, I can see myself easily working another 10 years because I want to."

Chris L. 54-year-old male

WHAT'S DIFFERENT ABOUT ACCELERATE WELLNESS?

Accelerate Wellness is the result of over two decades of researching, testing, and fine-tuning a process that is simple and fool-proof; follow the steps, trust the process, and you will get results. This guarantee is possible because of the following key differentiators that define the Accelerate Wellness approach:

One: First Things First. Everyone has that friend who went on a crash diet (or maybe you did yourself). Keto, South Beach, Paleo, Jenny Craig, or any of dozens of other plans. They lose a ton of weight very quickly, toss all their old clothes, and resolve never to regain the weight again. But within a few months, we all know what happens: As soon as they go off the strict regimen, the weight comes back — sometimes bringing more with it!

Why does this happen? One huge reason is that the changes were unsustainable. As soon as the external structure of the prescribed diet is removed, willpower isn't enough to keep the weight off. The individual needs to address the mindset issues that may have contributed to an environment of stress, overeating, or toxicity.

Another reason is that the body itself hasn't truly healed. There may be deficiencies at the cellular level that have impacted metabolism, and that means eating even what might be considered a "healthy" diet will never support a lower body weight because there are key issues that need to be addressed to restore the person's body to healthy functioning. Insulin resistance, for instance, can interfere with maintaining a healthy weight.

This phenomenon isn't limited to weight loss, though that's a readily understandable example because it tends to be visible. But think about the same thing with diabetes. If you're diagnosed as diabetic or pre-diabetic, a change in nutrition may be enough to lower your blood sugar so you are no longer in the danger zone. But if the second you get a clean bill of health, you return to snacks of Snickers and meals centered on refined carbs and sugar, you're most likely going to end up in the same place. Deeper changes must be put in place in order to achieve longer-lasting change.

That's why Accelerate Wellness focuses on first things first. The first step is detoxifying the body, followed by replacing those toxins with nutrients. This is also the time to begin the process of creating healthy habits and a mindset that will support these changes so you're truly healing for life. The whole process is designed to take you through and smoothly integrate a full-body wellness protocol.

Two: Essentialism. There are an unlimited number of actions you can take to improve your mental and physical health. It seems like every day there's a new exercise, supplement, or approach to fitness that is guaranteed to lower cholesterol, combat disease, trim your waistline, or help you sleep better. But trying to incorporate all of these various recommendations into your life is impossible. And, in fact, many of these possibilities, ideas, and activities sound great and seem important, but serve no significant purpose — or can actually work counter to long-term health and wellbeing.

When you're busy trying to do too much at once, you end up burnt out, overwhelmed, and discouraged. That's because you end up giving partial effort to many things, instead of full effort to the critical few. That's why the Accelerate Wellness program was designed through the lens of essentialism, which means focusing only on the elements that actually contribute to the goal you're trying to achieve. It's the 80/20 Rule in action: By concentrating on the elements that truly move the needle, you will end up reaching your goals more efficiently and effectively.

By adopting an essentialist view of health, the elements you need to reset your health and prepare for perpetual healing have been clearly identified. Everything you are asked to do along the way in the seven months of the Accelerate Wellness program is a critical part of the process. When you take part in Accelerate Wellness, you know you're focusing on the 20 percent of activities, habits, and behaviors that will bring the results you desire. And once you start getting results, you'll create momentum to keep moving forward.

Peptides — discussed in greater depth in chapter 4 — are part of the essential few that will make a huge difference in your health. (Note: if you'd like to read more about the philosophy of essentialism, check out the book, *Essentialism: The Disciplined Pursuit of Less,* by Greg McKeown).

Three: Never Stop Healing. When you take part in the Accelerate Wellness program, you're creating habits and behaviors that will help you in the present with linear results, but you're also investing in your future. The goal is not just to "fix" deficiencies so you feel better now, but to create lifelong health and wellness.

It's different from going on a crash diet to lose weight to fit into an outfit for your 30th high school reunion or your daughter's wedding. It may help out in the short term, but once you stop the behavior, you're back where you started. Most of western medicine is focused on linear results like this: you have high blood pressure, you take medication, your blood pressure comes down. But that's not long-term health.

Accelerate Wellness is not interested in short-term fixes. The program is about healing from your very cells outward, creating residual outcomes, meaning a decade from now you're thanking yourself for the investments you made in your health today. With Accelerate Wellness, you're creating a foundation of health that will serve you for years to come.

Your Turn

What does optimal health mean to you?

_____

_____

_____

_____

_____

_____

_____

_____

_____

Jot down a few thoughts about what you'd like your life to look like 10 years from now. What do you think you'll need to change now to bring about that ideal future?

_____

_____

_____

_____

_____

_____

_____

_____

_____

_____

_____

_____

_____

_____

CHAPTER 4

THE "MAGIC" OF PEPTIDES

Before getting into the specifics of each stage of the Accelerate Wellness program, the following is a cursory overview into the "secret sauce" that makes this seven-month program so successful: peptides.

> **Note:** Even if you're tempted to skip this chapter, please at least skim it. It's critical for you to understand a bit about the history, structure, and use of peptides, so you'll understand why they're such an integral part of our Accelerate Wellness Program. Reading this chapter will take just a few minutes, and it will give you a whole new appreciation for the beauty and science of your body!

Peptides have become a leading therapy at East West Health because they bring so many benefits with them. First, they don't tend to have toxic accumulation based on their short half-life. Contrast that with some supplements, such as fat-soluble vitamins, which can accumulate in the body and potentially lead to toxicity and harmful side effects.[5]

Second, they are safe when combined with other pharmaceuticals and supplements, which isn't always the case with other medications and supplements — even so-called "natural" ones. Combining dietary supplements and medications could result in dangerous interactions. For instance, the effects of some drugs, such as birth control pills and treatments for depression and heart disease, can be compromised when taken with St. John's wort, an herbal supplement.[6] This isn't the case with peptides.

Next, it has been shown that peptides increase a healing response two to three times faster than diet, lifestyle, and supplements alone. (Note: this isn't always the case. When used with incongruent lifestyles, peptides can have a lesser impact on the physiological or physiological conditions of our patients.)

Safety, speed, and efficacy. Now that it's clear why working with peptides is effective, it is time get into what they are.

WHAT IS A PEPTIDE?

As with any medical or health-related topic, it can be difficult to isolate exactly what peptides are and how they work because they're built into many other processes and functions in the body. In the interests of keeping this topic manageable, the following presents a simplified approach (if you'd like to learn more or go deeper, I suggest you listen to the Accelerate Wellness podcast, available wherever you like to listen, or at https://acueastwest.com/). A simple definition is that peptides are the building blocks of proteins and are composed of amino acids that work to regulate a variety of biological functions and processes. These naturally occurring peptides act as signaling molecules within the body and instruct other cells and molecules on what functions to perform.

The following unpacks that a little more so you can see why they're so effective, and why they are a cornerstone of the Accelerate Wellness program.

As you may remember from high school biology, every cell in your body contains proteins, which are strings of organic molecules (meaning they contain carbon) that make up all of your organs and systems. Diving down another level, proteins in turn comprise hundreds or even thousands of individual amino acids.

Peptides are small-chain amino acids, made up of no more than fifty acids. Over 7,000 known peptide types are produced naturally in your body, and they influence different functions in the body, such as better hormone production or cell regulation.

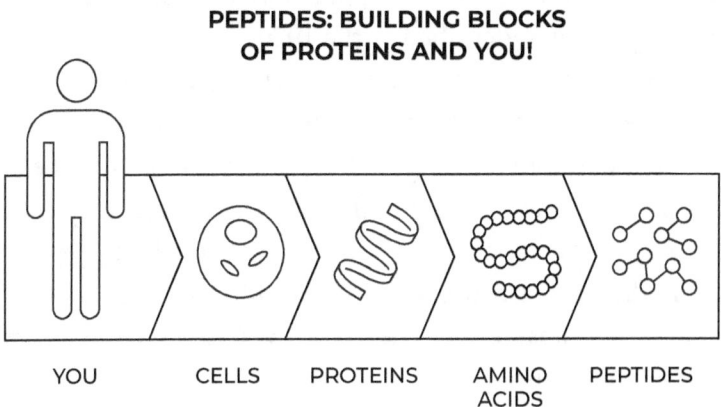

PEPTIDES: BUILDING BLOCKS OF PROTEINS AND YOU!

YOU   CELLS   PROTEINS   AMINO ACIDS   PEPTIDES

Of the 7,000-plus peptides we know about, only a small number — about 500 total — have been sequenced and are available for therapeutic purposes, including growth factors, anti-infective agents, neurotransmitters, hormones, and more.[7] This is an exciting field of research, with new discoveries being made all the time.

WHERE DID THEY COME FROM?

In 1986, an explosion rocked the nuclear reactor in Chernobyl, Ukraine, leaking huge amounts of radiation into the atmosphere and contaminating the entire area. In order to stop the casualties, Dr. Vladimir Khavinson, a specialist in treatment and prevention, was tapped to prevent cancer in emergency responders. "People who used the products for their immune system, the brain, their reproductive system, have a longer life span and fewer cases of cancer," Dr. Khavinson recalls.[8] The products he's referring to? Mini-protein structures called peptides, small amino acids that help regulate cell division and genetic expression, that Dr. Khavinson and his team first identified in the 1970s.

These peptides play a foundational role in repairing every tissue, organ, and gland in the body. His team discovered that peptides are signaling molecules that bind like a Lego to receptors on the surface of the cell. Once there, they activate a genetic response that allows cells to function properly again. They express disease and turn off sickness. The body has amazing capabilities to heal when you express the correct healing mechanisms.

Since Khavinson's discoveries, the worldwide medical community has made great strides in identification, sequencing, and of peptides for health, wellness, and treatment of disease.

CLEANING UP THE BODY'S PROCESSES

One way to describe how peptides help your body reset, restore, and recharge itself is with the metaphor of a copy machine. Imagine you make a single black-and-white copy of a sheet of text. Then you take the copy, and copy it. Again, you take the copy and copy it. Do that over and over and over a thousand times, and what happens? The copy loses its integrity and becomes less clear. Keep going, and the output will eventually become unreadable.

Now imagine that copying process took place not 1,000 times... not 10,000 times... but TWO TRILLION TIMES, each and every day. That's what happens to the 3 billion digits in the DNA, in each of your cells as it divides and "copies" itself.[9]

Peptides work by mimicking the same expression that your body is already utilizing, and "cleaning up" the communication package in your cells, making your bodily functions more effective and bringing you to new levels of wellness. Peptides work "epigenetically", meaning they turn off genes that manifest disease and turn on longevity promoting genes. Peptides jumpstart the healing process because they interact with hundreds of healing pathways in the body, which is also why they work quicker than most therapies.

Peptide therapy is a treatment method that stimulates cellular regrowth systems. Because they are made up of short amino acid chains, they are able to attach to receptors on the surface of cells. This allows them to provide cells and molecules with instructions for specific actions. Peptides are critical to facilitating body responses and actions, and they can be beneficial for treatments of specific concerns safely and effectively.

As you learn about the role of peptides, you may start thinking about hormones and how they perform similar functions — and in a sense, you'd be right. A simple definition of a hormone is a chemical substance that acts like a "messenger molecule" in the body, helping to control how cells and organs function.[10] If you were asked to name some hormones, you could probably do so readily: insulin, testosterone, DHEA, progesterone… they all act by binding with a receptor site and instigating a particular function.

But what happens when your hormones are out of whack, due to changes in the body (like menopause) or to outside forces (like from our food or from medication)? When that happens, your body's ability to produce the hormones it needs to function properly can be compromised. For instance, it's common for a menopausal woman to be placed on progesterone and estrogen. Unfortunately, that can actually downregulate her ability to make the proper hormones, further exacerbating her symptoms.

That's where peptides come in. They clean up that message so this woman's body, specifically the endocrine system, actually receives the signal to start producing hormones, allowing her body to do its job.

WHY PEPTIDES?

One of the questions commonly asked is, "Why do I need peptides? I have a great diet. I mainly eat whole foods. I get a lot of exercise. Can't I just take some herbs or something?"

The short answer is yes, you could take herbs or supplements, and you could also increase your consumption of foods with peptides, such as soy, meats, flaxseed, or hemp seeds. But if you need to get from Point A to Point B on a map, do you want to take the slow roads that are full of traffic and bad weather patterns, or do you want to hop on the expressway? The supplement way can get you at least part of the way to your destination, but peptides shorten the healing time. If you're truly concerned about your health, you probably want to get there as soon as possible.

And if you're in pain, or you are suffering, you can accelerate healing with peptides.

Another reason peptides are superior to supplementation is the potency. The amount of supplementation you'd have to take to match the power and effectiveness of peptides could be insurmountable in terms of cost and volume. Peptides are much more effective, making them more cost-effective as well.

For some people, supplementation isn't possible. For instance, if you have a bacterial infection, or you are having digestive issues — and approximately 40 percent of American adults have some kind of functional gut issue[11] — you might not be able to break down the supplements. Then you're simply taking them and eliminating them, generating very expensive urine and excrement.

Conversely, because most peptides are injected (don't get squeamish — it's a very small insulin needle that most people do not feel), they bypass the digestive system and the metabolic process is very simple. Not only do most of the peptides bypass the typical digestive barriers that can keep them from being absorbed, they activate the entire body through cell-to-cell communication so that the area in distress gets the signal instantly, which leads to rapid accelerations in healing.

THE BOTTOM LINE

In sum, peptides are an integral part of most biological processes and are present throughout every cell and tissue in the body. Maintenance of appropriate concentration and activity levels of peptides is necessary to achieve homeostasis and maintain health. The function of a peptide is determined by its size and amino acid sequence.

Peptides are smaller molecules than proteins or antibody medications and bind to their cellular targets more selectively than chemical drugs or natural supplements that must be broken down sufficiently by the digestive system.

Because they hit the cellular targets more effectively than drugs or supplements, peptides have very few adverse side effects. Peptides don't set off an immune alarm or histamine response.

As mentioned above, of the 7,000-plus peptides naturally occurring in the human body, only about 500 have been sequenced, and about 100 have been studied and approved by the FDA to treat one or more diseases. Others are available as dietary supplements (which, for the reasons mentioned above, are typically not ideal), orally, through nasal sprays, or by injection.

Peptides derived from food sources and turned into oral supplements are sold over-the-counter. You might be familiar with collagen peptides, which you can find at a grocery or health food store, but the gold standard of peptides are available by prescription.

Like many medications that are available on the black market, so are peptides, although purchasing them outside of a prescription with a knowledgeable medical provider can increase your risks. You may decrease your costs, but what most non-regulated peptide sources are giving you are fragments of the entire peptide complex, which can diminish the results. By some estimates, "80 percent of the peptides advertised on the web are adulterated or outright fakes," according to Michael Powell in an article for the *New York Times*.[12]

The Accelerate Wellness program only uses peptides from carefully vetted, 503a and 503b regulated compounding pharmacies like Wells Pharmacy, because of their safety standards and quality controls. Each peptide prescription goes through a medical team review and audit.

Peptides have very low to no toxic effects and have proven safety records. They can easily be used simultaneously with other treatments like hormones, medications, and herbs with almost no contraindications. Many peptides can be given up to a 100x greater dose than medication without any known side effects. Increasing the peptide dose doesn't equate to a better therapeutic benefit because the body doesn't respond to what it doesn't need.

MAKING THE MOST OF PEPTIDES

Peptides work best when used with charged nutrients, particles, and gentle binders. These molecules create a better internal environment for peptides to communicate in because they change the pH of the body and facilitate a better energy exchange on the electron transport chain, which in turn advantageously influences the mitochondrial cell danger response.

Peptides are best used as a stack, meaning using more than one peptide to speed up the results, because together we've seen a multiplying effect. Peptides are also best used to open pathways and not to treat symptoms or diseases. Most doctors practice reductionist medicine and fail to fully see the capabilities of peptides because they are more closely watching the progression of disease and symptoms. Peptides best serve the body by turning on genetic information so that your body can go back to its "factory installed" healing capabilities as the rust is dusted off the healthy genes so that they can express vitality.

This is only at the cusp of peptide therapy, and every month there's new breakthrough research that provides greater awareness of the science of peptides.

WHAT ARE THEY GOOD FOR?

The unique property of peptides can be harnessed and used to treat specific conditions through peptide therapy.

Peptides can be:

Transporters – like glucose transporters that are necessary for glucose to travel from the blood into the muscle.

Enzymes – biological catalysts that speed up metabolic reactions. Most of the hundreds of enzymes are peptides.

Hormones – biological messengers that carry information from one tissue through the blood to a distant tissue. Two common classes of hormones are peptide and steroid hormones. Examples of peptide hormones include those involved in blood glucose regulation, such as insulin and glucagon and those that regulate appetites, such as ghrelin and leptin.

Structural components – peptides like actin and myosin function as structural elements of the muscle, and some other peptides contribute to bone shape and strength.

Here are a few ways peptide therapy is used:

- accelerate healing processes
- boost hormone levels
- build muscle mass
- decrease joint and muscle pain
- enhance cognitive function and memory
- increase levels of energy, stamina, and strength
- improve sleep quality
- lower blood pressure
- promote healthy immune function
- reduce signs of aging
- stimulate hair growth
- help reverse symptoms of sexual dysfunction

The most exciting science of peptides is the fact that they are pleiotropic by nature. Pleiotropic means that they produce more than one effect or have multiple phenotypic expressions of a pleiotropic gene.

Pleiotropy occurs when one gene influences two or more seemingly unrelated phenotypic traits. Such a gene that exhibits multiple phenotypic expressions is called a pleiotropic gene. This is one of the primary reasons that the Accelerate Wellness program starts with six initial months of peptides combined to open targeted pathways in the body for maximizing therapeutic responses, mitochondrial health, and removing interferences in the body.

> **Resource:** An overview of some of the most commonly used peptides is included in Appendix A at the end of this book.

OKAY, WHICH ONES DO I NEED?

Although we're all made of the same essential ingredients, how each person's body functions is entirely unique. We can talk in generalities about what you *might* need, but self-diagnosis can be a dangerous thing. What you think is going on in your body might not actually be the real issue, as symptoms can be caused by multiple root causes. That's why before any person commits to the Accelerate Wellness program, the first step is a blood panel. This provides the information necessary to be able to diagnose a precise protocol for you. Each of the three phases of the Accelerate Wellness program have different goals, and it's critical to approach each in order, in a manner that's specifically designed for you and your health goals.

Now that you understand what peptides are and how they work in the body to fight disease, reverse the effects of aging, and increase wellness, it is time to see how they're used in the Accelerate Wellness program.

Your Turn

Was there any information in this chapter that surprised you about peptides?

_____

_____

_____

_____

_____

_____

Which aspect of peptides is most appealing to you? (select all that apply):

- Safety

- Effectiveness

- Potential uses

- Helps my body heal itself

- Additional aspects that are appealing:

_____

_____

_____

_____

CHAPTER 5

DEEP DIVE: RESET

Now that you have an overview of the Accelerate Wellness program and what makes this approach different, it is time to take a look at your first 60 days as you Reset your body.

As discussed in chapter 3, optimal health depends on optimal cell-to-cell communication. If your cells are unable to communicate effectively due to interferences, deficiencies, or inflammation, your mitochondria (the cell's energy motor) senses a problem and activates an immune response called cell danger response, or CDR. The CDR is your body's attempt to protect itself, but in doing so, it interrupts normal function and can produce changes in hormone production, cellular electron flow, oxygen consumption, bioenergetics, and more.[13]

That's why the first step to wellness is to Reset your cells for ideal cell-to-cell communication. Think of it like resetting your computer or smartphone when things go awry; by restoring normal functioning, you can get your electronic devices — and your body — working as intended.

In the Reset phase (days 1-60), you are beginning the process of transforming every cell in your body, removing interferences and biotoxins, and turning on amazing cell-to-cell communication.

Here's what your Reset phase includes:

- **Core Daily Actions.** The daily "6 Essentials" that will support your progress during that phase. You'll be asked to score yourself each day on how many of these you meet.

- **Phase-Specific Peptides.** The highest quality of peptides available to assist you in bypassing many of the cellular, genetic, and mitochondrial issues that might keep you from advancing. They are specifically selected for each phase and are chosen for their safety, effectiveness, and clinical outcomes.

- **CellCore Detox Supplements.** CellCore Biosciences is the industry leader in digestive, immune, and mitochondrial health. Their customized protocols will help you restore effective cellular communication. Their products are available only through qualified health practitioners.

- **Additional Supportive Peptides.** In addition to the phase-specific peptides, additional peptides may be recommended for your unique needs.

What You May Experience:

The Reset phase is the foundational stage for you to make significant lifestyle changes. Most patients notice that they instantly have a reduction in digestive issues, such as bloating. They feel like their body is more aligned with their spirit.

They sleep better. And by far, the biggest benefit stated over and over is that their energy is off the charts. Many times they say they can't believe how quickly their energy levels increase because it's been so long since they've actually felt good. If you've been in pain, you should notice a reduction in discomfort.

While weight loss is not the focus of this phase, it's not uncommon for you to begin to lose stored fat — sometimes very quickly — as your body begins to heal. Even patients who feel like they've tried every diet under the sun are surprised at how fast the weight comes off when they make the needed lifestyle changes.

"I'm golfing again!"

Total knee replacement was imminent, but six months ago I decided to apply for the Accelerate Wellness program at East West Health. I can now climb stairs again without any problem, I am playing golf and going about my normal life again. I am very satisfied with the results I got and would recommend East West Health to anyone experiencing pain and lack of mobility. I would do it again tomorrow.

Gary D., 62-year-old male

The downside to the 60-day reset is that you might feel frustrated without knowing what to eat or exactly how and when to exercise, you might even feel a bit restless the first few nights as you are getting to bed earlier. Even increasing your hydration can be challenging on the days that you forget to bring your favorite non-plastic water bottle on your day's adventures. But as you read on and learn about the 6 Reset Essentials, you are encouraged to try them out for yourself and see if you don't find another 10 or even 20 percent greater levels of energy.

"Much easier than I expected!"

Getting started with the Reset protocol was much easier than I expected it to be. My downfall is sugar, and I thought I would never kick the habit of wanting something sweet after meals. Regan and his team assured me that the peptides would help curb the cravings... and they worked like magic! I made it 60 days with no sugar and have no intention of going back. I also noticed a big improvement in my strength and endurance on my hikes.

Bev, 72-year-old female

How It All Works Together	
Each phase of the Accelerate Wellness program includes:	**Additionally, when you work with the Accelerate Wellness team, your experience is enhanced with:**
• Core Daily Actions	• Discovery Day, Orientation, and thorough lab testing
• Peptides for the Month's Focus	• Individualized accountability and support
• CellCore Detox Supplements	• Weekly group training
• Additional Supportive Peptides	• Support from fitness advisors, health coaches, and functional medicine providers

Core Daily Actions

After almost two decades of gathering clinical data with real people who are in a natural environment (not a blinded-placebo-non-reality study), six essential actions have been identified that move you towards your dream health in the most efficient ways possible. Each of the three Accelerate Wellness phases includes six core daily actions — defined as your "6 Essentials" — that will support your progress during that particular phase.

Think of these as your launchpad to great health that you can incorporate into your daily activities with some simple planning. In the Reset phase, these 6 Essentials will supercharge your energy and pull you out of pain quickly. They also help create lasting residual results that your future self will thank you for!

1. **Sleeping (9:30 PM to 5:30 AM).** You can survive longer without food than you can without sleep! Just a few nights without sleep and you'll experience hallucinations, cognitive impairment, and more.[14] Your body needs this time to relax, rebuild damaged tissues, and reduce inflammatory states. By falling asleep before 10 PM, you will activate growth hormones and turn off the aging process.

   Tips for a good night's sleep: Eat your last meal three hours before bed, and avoid screens like TVs, computers, or phones an hour before bed. Using blue-light blockers on your screens or wearing blue-light blocking glasses will also help filter out the artificial light that tricks your brain into thinking it's still daytime. Reading, stretching, and meditating can all help you prepare for sleep. Other suggestions: Set the thermostat to 70 degrees, get a good air purifier, and tape your mouth shut if you snore (and get tested for sleep apnea ASAP!).

2. **Hydration.** When you wake up in the morning, you're already 8-12 oz dehydrated (which is why your brain may be fuzzy), so kick off your day with a glass of water. Your muscles and brain are the first regions to get dehydrated, which can lead to sore muscles and brain fog. Your goal is half your bodyweight in ounces of filtered or spring water — minimum! To jazz up your water, add some lemon and a pinch of salt or some Redmond's electrolyte blends without sugar.

The Downside of Hydration

One of our program participants had a specific complaint about all the water he was drinking in the Reset phase: He was waking up four times a night to urinate! Fortunately, this drawback has a very simple solution: Finish your last glass of water at least two hours before bedtime. When he made that switch, he was suddenly getting the best sleep of his life!

---

3. **<1 g Sugar.** No matter how good it tastes, sugar is not your friend. Sugar can destroy joint health, increase oxidative (heart) stress, and leave your gut exposed

to more infections. 70-100g of sugar can put your immune system into a coma-like state![15] Look at the labels of what you're eating, or better yet, eat only food that doesn't come in a package, contains no artificial ingredients, and is as close to organic and wild as possible.

Sugar Ain't All Sweet

Most people don't realize how much sugar they're eating! I have people who swear up and down that they eat very little sugar. "I don't have a sweet tooth," they say. "I don't eat any sugar at all!" Then they start tracking their food and they're shocked at the amount of sugar they're consuming without knowing it. Making the shift to reading labels and not eating anything with more than a gram of sugar per serving can drastically change your palate. You'll quickly notice your sugar cravings disappear.

---

4. **Exercise 30/30.** Move your body at least 60 minutes per day. Ideally, get outside for 30 minutes for a sunrise or sunset walk, bike, or hike. Push harder on the days you feel up to it, and gently ease into it on the days you don't. Spend the additional 30 minutes lifting heavy things — yes, your 3-year-old counts! You can also opt for yoga, pilates, Tabata or HIIT (high-intensity interval training). Just do it every day.

5. **Cold + Heat Exposure.** Your body has both heat and cold shock proteins, both of which are activated by heat and cold exposure. These proteins keep your mitochondria healthy and energy-efficient while you

shiver and sweat. Just two minutes in a cold shower helps calm your stress hormones, tighten skin, and trigger your belly fat to be burned for heat. If you like, you can model Wim Hoff and jump into an ice bath. Treat yourself to the opposite, too, with a 15 - 20 minute bath with Epsom salts (candlelight and Celine Dion on your phone are optional).

6. **Mindset Morning.** When you own the morning, you own the day. The Mindset Morning is your core habit that will lead to all the other habits. Here's how it goes:

- Upon waking, start your day by enjoying a glass of electrolyte-infused water.

- Set a timer for two minutes of deep breathing (this is a great time to focus on your life and health).

- Set the timer for another two minutes and focus on your future self: "I am alert, fit, pain-free, active, happy, giving, wise, fun, loving, etc." Think of someone you can do an act of kindness for today, and set a reminder to do so.

- Set the timer for another two minutes. Go through each of the "6 Essentials" to remind yourself of what you need to prioritize throughout your day.

- Keep track of your progress as you accomplish your "6 Essentials."

The 60-Day Progress Report

Score yourself each day one out of six for the number of healthy habits you participated in. Give yourself bonus points for going above and beyond light and learning a new skill, meal prep, taking peptides, and sell corn detox.

Each day, on a scale of 1 to 6, score yourself on participating in each of the 6 Essentials.

TOTAL POSSIBLE POINTS 360	YOUR SCORE:

Day 0-30: Hypothalamus / Pituitary / Adrenal (HPA) Axis Reset

The *hypothalamus* is the part of your brain that produces hormones that control:

- Body temperature
- Heart rate
- Hunger
- Mood
- Release of hormones from many glands, especially the pituitary gland
- Sex drive
- Sleep
- Thirst

When it is not operating correctly, you can experience increased appetite and rapid weight gain, low body temperature, slow heart rate, and a number of other issues.[16]

Connected by a stalk to the hypothalamus, the *pituitary gland* produces hormones that monitor and regulate bodily functions such as:

- Growth and sexual/reproductive development and function
- Glands (thyroid gland, adrenal glands, and gonads)
- Organs (kidneys, uterus, and breasts)

The pituitary gland is connected by a stalk to the hypothalamus. Together, the brain and pituitary gland form the neuroendocrine system.[17]

The *adrenal glands*, located on top of both kidneys, produce hormones that help regulate many essential bodily functions such as your metabolism, immune system, blood pressure, stress response, and more.[18]

These three are referred to as your HPA Axis, which regulates a number of physiological processes in your body, such as metabolism, immune responses, and the autonomic nervous system.[19]

The HPA Axis Reset allows new programming to support the brain/nervous system, hormones, gut, and circadian rhythms. Emotional, physical, infections, and chemicals — known as "EPIC" — stress patterns interfere with proper signaling in the body. It's easy to see how critical it is for your HPA Axis to be in top shape. The primary focus of the first 30 days of this phase is on eliminating interference and supporting proper functioning.

Day 0-30: Peptides

The core peptides to influence these pathways are:

- **Epitalon.** It works on the HPA Axis by activating the *pineal gland*, which is located in the center of the brain and produces and secretes melatonin, which can calm the adrenal response and stabilize the parasympathetic nervous symptom.

- **Selank.** It increases Gamma-Aminobutyric acid (GABA) while calming brain inflammation. It also has its own anti-microbial properties and stabilizes auto-immune pathways in the central nervous system.

> ### "I slept seven hours straight!"
>
> "I haven't had more than three hours of uninterrupted sleep in the past decade, and after my first injection of Epitalon, I slept seven hours straight! Three months later, I'm shocked at the great sleep I enjoy. Thank you Regan!!!"
>
> *Patty D., 58-year-old female*

Day 0-30: CellCore Detox Supplements

The high-quality supplements to support these pathways are:

- **Energy and Drainage.** Detoxification relies on adequate passage of waste, so we're focusing on opening your filtration and drainage.

- **Tauroursodeoxycholic acid (TUDCA).** A bile salt that enhances liver and digestive function and supports Phase 1 and Phase II liver detox, as well as liver drainage (sometimes called Phase III). It also encourages glutathione synthesis to provide antioxidant support.

- **CT-Minerals.** A liquid supplement that supplies minerals and amino acids to support routine detoxification. It also promotes cellular uptake at any pH level due to its formulation with fulvic acid extracts, and it provides building blocks for cellular energy production, which is needed for detoxification.

- **BioToxin Binder.** Promotes the body's natural ability to detoxify by binding and removing ammonia and other unwanted microbial byproducts. It also supports sulfur pathways, which help maintain normal sensitivity levels. It promotes oxygen production in the body, and nurtures a healthy gut microbiome.

- **KL Support (Kidney/Liver).** Healthy kidney and liver function is essential to good health. This supports fat metabolism, hepatic blood flow, and healthy urinary tract and bladder function, while helping the body carry out its natural detoxification processes.

- **Bowel Mover.** A natural digestive aid that encourages soft bowel movements, supports intestinal health, peristalsis, and proper digestive function.

Day 31-60: Mindy/Body Growth Hormone (GH) Recovery

Growth hormone (GH) is produced by the pituitary gland. Not only does it fuel growth in childhood and adolescence, it also helps maintain tissues and organs throughout life. Beginning in middle age, the pituitary gland slowly reduces the amount of GH it produces.[20]

In this phase, the focus is to activate the GH pathway by removing interference and inflammation, and boosting energy levels. You're now building new skeletal muscle, restoring liver function, increasing cardiovascular fitness, and improving cognition. Your entire endocrine system (thyroid, adrenals, hypothalamus, pituitary, and pineal gland) are being optimized so that estrogens, testosterone, progesterone, and thyroid hormones all turn on again.

Day 31-60 Peptides

The core peptides to influence these pathways are:

- **CJC1295/Ipamorelin.** These GH-releasing peptides have been shown to diminish sugar cravings, convert fat into muscle, and restore the liver after damage.

- **Thymosin Beta 4:** This regenerative peptide will prevent muscle soreness from lactic acid build-up. It assists in faster recovery after your new workouts.

Day 31-60 CellCore Detox

The high-quality supplements to support gut and immune for removal of parasites and microbes are:

- **Para 1.** Acts as a "gut grabber," forming a sticky mass and binding unwanted factors. It facilitates detox protocols and supports health in maintenance programs.

- **Para 2.** Supports the body's natural mechanism for removing unwanted factors. Promotes digestive tract health, including normal bile flow, microbiome composition, and bowel movements. It also nurtures the body's immune and antioxidant systems, aiding inflammatory balance.

- **VidRadChem Binder.** Supports immune cell activity, inflammatory balance, and microbiome health. Offers an optimal blend of herbs in a tincture format to maximize potency. Provides phytochemicals to support liver and digestive health.

- **KL Support (Kidney/Liver).** Healthy kidney and liver function is essential to good health. This supports fat metabolism, hepatic blood flow, and healthy urinary tract and bladder function, while helping the body carry out its natural detoxification processes.

Phase 1: Additional Peptides That May Be Recommended for You:

- **BPC-157 PURE.** The Body Protective Complex (BPC) peptide activates the healing of the joints, digestive barriers, and muscle tissue. Helps with leaky gut, digestive issues, and liver health.

- **Thymosin Beta 4.** This peptide allows the body to build new blood vessels. It promotes stem cell heath and repairs the endothelial cells for cardio health. It's known as a "master peptide" to reset the immune system for autoimmune issues. Not only does it promote systemic healing, it also improves wound healing and repair throughout the body, including not only the skin, but the brain, spinal cord, and heart. This peptide travels easily throughout the body, which promotes faster healing. Can be injected at the site of injury for an improved outcome.

- **Sarcotropin.** This peptide includes ingredients for fat metabolism, recovery, muscle growth, increased energy and sleep support, gut, cardiovascular, and hormonal health, bone density, memory and cognitive performance, focus, increased blood flow and arterial repair, appetite suppression and improved digestion.

- **GHK-CU.** These copper peptides recruit stem cells into damaged areas and build greater collagen and connective tissue. Reduces wrinkles and increases vascularity.

Weight Loss Peptides:

- **MOTS-c (Mitochondrial booster).** Correcting the mitochondrial function will keep your metabolic engine running cleanly while elevating your energy levels. Research shows that MOTS-c helps stabilize glucose sensitivity, prevents weight gain, and optimizes muscle repair.

- **5-amino-1MQ.** Increases athletic performance and maximizes recovery. 5-amino-1MQ also activates the AMPk pathway for greater muscle adaptability and improves flexibility while turning fat into muscle.

- **Tesofensine.** Tesofensine has shown to be incredibly helpful for weight loss by increasing serotonin, which helps with food cravings. It also improves dopamine, making you satiated faster for less overeating, and increases epinephrine, which allows you to burn fat more efficiently.

- **Semaglutide.** Clinical trials show Semaglutide to be nearly as effective as a bariatric bypass surgery or a lap band without the risks of surgery. It's one of the best peptides to use for sugar cravings and lowers blood sugar.[21]

CHAPTER 6

DEEP DIVE: RECHARGE

Congratulations on completion of your first phase! Forging new habits and creating new levels of health is not always easy, so make sure to give yourself credit. By now, you should be feeling (and most likely seeing) some of the results of your work

The biggest objective in Phase 1: 60-Day Reset was to remove interferences and inflammation so that your body can detoxify and heal. Your body now has better detoxification capabilities, your stress-response axis (HPA Axis) is no longer on tilt, and you can enjoy greater levels of energy and clarity in your life.

Our next phase (Phase 2, days 61-120) concentrates on your DNA, gut health, and mitochondria as you continue the journey to optimal cell-to-cell communication. You're going to be putting energy back into every organ, gland, and cell in your body. There's a saying in the Tao Te Ching, "To know enough's enough is enough to know." The Phase 2: 60-Day Recharge is focused on energy and momentum and on helping you to stay calm and clear while you move towards your greater future self.

Think of the first two phases as you would a computer system. Phase 1: Reset, was optimizing your hardware, rebooting and reseting everything to factory settings so any software you install will work properly. Now, the Recharge phase is about transforming and updating your software.

One exciting thing about the Recharge phase is you begin to get residual, versus linear, outcomes. A linear benefit is where you take an antibiotic and you get rid of an infection. A residual benefit is where you use a peptide like Epitalon and you turn on different genetic pathways, so now your body can start to have long-lasting results. The Recharge phase is essentially like turning your batteries back on. It's like charging up an electric car so it can go more miles with more speed and more enjoyment.

You will be doing a systemic detox with CellCore and opening up metabolic pathways, increasing the digestive enzymes in the body so there's better gastric secretions and healing the gut.

Here's What Your Recharge Phase Includes:

- **Core Daily Actions.** The daily "6 Essentials" that will support your progress during that phase. You will be asked to score yourself each day on how many of the essentials you meet.

- **Phase-Specific Peptides.** The highest quality of peptides available to assist you in bypassing many of the cellular, genetic, and mitochondrial issues that might keep you from advancing. They are specifically selected for each phase, and are chosen for their safety, effectiveness, and clinical outcomes.

- **CellCore Detox Supplements.** CellCore Biosciences is the industry leader in digestive, immune, and mitochondrial health. Their customized protocols will help you restore effective cellular communication. Many of the CellCore products use the unique Carbon Technology through a blend of fulvic acids and polysaccharides that support cellular repair and the body's natural ability to detoxify. With a low pH, Carbon Technology also helps protect ingredients from being digested by stomach acid, so that they remain intact as they enter the desired location in the body. Carbon Technology may very well transform the supplement industry in the next decade. A special recipe is used to allow for better signaling of your peptide pathways. Their products are available only through qualified health practitioners.

What You May Experience: In this phase, people notice a massive change in their energy. It's like turning the lights on in your cells, and it's getting your mitochondria prepared for the next phase so that your mitochondria can now start to produce more energy with less effort.

It is also a powerful time because now you're maximizing your body's ability to eliminate waste in all three phases of detoxification. You'll notice that you have less puffiness in your neck and around your legs. Additionally, many patients notice an extreme change in their waist circumference, leading to a trip to the shopping mall because their body has changed quite substantially from the Reset phase. Now, Recharge is when muscles start to show up that haven't been there for a long time. One patient very excitedly reported that the change he noticed most is the ability to lift heavy objects with half of the effort. He was thrilled because he can take care of his farm better, he can play with his grandkids with more vigor, and he just feels better about life in general by being stronger.

Another patient in this phase said that the biggest thing she noticed was that her knees feel stronger, and her leg muscles are developing. After a skiing injury, she hadn't been able to do lunges in months, but she just couldn't develop the quad muscle that she had before the injury. Now that she's on the appropriate peptides and she's following the detoxification protocol, her leg muscles are more developed now, and so her knees feel stronger and more stable.

A lot of people also notice that their libido spikes. One couple — the woman is in her 50s and he is in his 60s — experienced this change and acted super giggly with each other. They reported that they have had more intimacy in the last few weeks than they've had in the last 20 years of their marriage because of the way that they feel on the program!

The second part of the Recharge phase is about gut health. A comprehensive stool test is conducted to determine if there's any inflammation in the gut, looking at all the bacteria to see if there's any undergrowth or overgrowth of pathogenic bacteria and if there are any infections. Enzymatic production in the gut is assessed as well.

In addition to getting the gut healthy, you will detox from heavy metals, activate hormones, and get your body muscle mass built up to create more athleticism. In addition to the reduced inflammation and puffiness and greater energy, your hair starts feeling thicker, and you're sleeping better.

"My energy has doubled!"

I've learned how to exercise in ways that I never thought I could. I'm breathing through my belly, which I've never been able to do. I had a virus 10 days ago, but I noticed I got through it faster than I ever remember getting through a cold. They used to set me back for about a month. I've increased my protein consumption. Now I'm eating an enormous amount, but I feel incredibly energized by it. My focus on hydration and fiber has also been a game changer. I'm sleeping better, and my energy has improved at least double. I've also noticed that my accountability to myself is so much more powerful, to the point I do not need that evening drink. I've made phenomenal improvements in the choices I'm making, in my stress levels, and in my ability to be a great mother and grandmother.

Christine, 67-year-old female

Core Daily Actions

Each of the three Accelerate Wellness phases includes six core daily actions — defined as your "6 Essentials" — that will support your progress during that phase. In the Recharge phase, these 6 Essentials will give you your health and your time back as we truly focus on what's *essential* for optimal health. Some amazing benefits come in the six essentials in the Recharge phase. As you can see, you are building on the habits you developed in the Reset phase, and layering on deeper levels of support for your liver, deeper support for your fitness levels and your muscles, and deeper support for athleticism and agility.

1. **Your Brain's Flow State.** Learning, novelty, and challenge set the stage for you to function at your peak. Finding yourself in a state of effortless action is what experts call the "flow state," a time when you are totally immersed in a task. Research shows that the brain secretes higher levels of the neurotransmitter dopamine when you are in flow.[22] Other benefits include enhanced performance and greater ability to concentrate for longer periods of time.[23]

   Play detective and find out what gets you into a flow state. It might be as simple as reading a good book or having a deep conversation, or you might also find your flow while speeding down the mountains on a capable bike or skis. Once you pinpoint your flow-generating activities, carve out time daily to enter this timeless space.

2. **Enjoyable Fitness.** Research shows that people who engage in 300 minutes of high-intensity physical activity or 600 minutes of moderate-intensity physical activity each week live up to 31% longer than those who do not.[24] With your 30/30 exercise habit in place from Phase 1: Reset, you are putting in the reps, but now make it enjoyable.

Think ahead a few decades. What are two or three activities that you'd like to still participate in at the age of 100? While there's no promise that you will be able to do those activities when you are 100, there is a promise that if you don't start now, and do them regularly, you won't! Incorporate one or more of these activities into your daily schedule.

3. **Build Muscle for Age Reversal.** Protein is the main macronutrient that's needed to keep you looking lean, strong, and fit in any decade of life. Your Recharge happens when you feed your body 1 gram of protein per pound of ideal body weight. If your goal is to weigh 200 lbs, then eat 200 grams of protein. If your body weight is ideal and you weigh 150 pounds, then eat 150 grams of supercharged, grass-fed, clean, healthy protein. Organ meats are especially beneficial for heart health, combating inflammation, fighting depression, and more.[25]

4. **Leak-Free Gut Zone.** Now that you've increased the protein in your diet, it's time to optimize gut health so that you can digest, absorb, and transport the amino acids you're consuming. Leaky gut, also called increased intestinal permeability, is a condition where the normally secure gut lining instead has cracks or holes, allowing everything from toxins to partially digested food to penetrate underlying tissues.[26] When

that happens, it triggers an inflammatory response that downregulates your ability to put protein to work. Sealing up the gut is best done by avoiding ibuprofen, gluten, emulsifiers, sugar, stress, A1 dairy casein proteins, and anything artificially sweetened or colored. Adding in either bone broth, colostrum, or collagen daily is your gut-zipping remedy.

5. **Love Your Liver Tender.** Turmeric, beets, arugula, and garlic are all liver-beneficial foods. Eating at least one of these a day will keep your liver healthy, your discernment sharp, and your resiliency legendary. Additionally, incorporate one protein fast day per week where you limit protein down to about 50 to 60 grams.

6. **Daily Pound of Vegetables.** I grew up in Idaho's Snake River Basin, so it's no surprise my mom had the ability to prepare potatoes more ways than I can count. While I'll never forsake my roots (pun intended), I learned to branch out from potatoes as my favorite vegetable. Your pound of veggies per day includes asparagus, chard, kale, broccolini, parsley, cilantro, leafy greens (lots), and anything else that catches your fancy in the produce section (or that you grow in your own garden). Be sure to steam or Insta-Pot your veggies for the best result and to eliminate any problematic oxalates or acids that your kidneys don't love.

The 60-Day Progress Report

Score yourself each day one out of six for the number of healthy habits you participated in. Give yourself bonus points for going above and beyond light and learning a new skill, meal prep, taking peptides, and sell corn detox.

Each day, on a scale of 1 to 6, score yourself on participating in each of the 6 Essentials.

TOTAL POSSIBLE POINTS 360	YOUR SCORE:

Phase 2: Peptides

The core peptides to influence these pathways are:

- **ARA290.** This is an amazing peptide for pain and for naturally increasing endorphins. Improves endurance and can even help with kidney issues.

- **LL37.** This recharge peptide assists in eradicating any microbial infections and can even penetrate sneaky biofilms that toxins can hide under. LL37 has cathelicidin properties and also repairs damage to the gut wall. When you combine LL37 with the peptide KPV, you get an even bigger boost in healing digestive issues that create bloating, gas, and brain fog.

- **BPC157.** BPC (Body Protective Complex) was first isolated from human gastric juices and has been shown to be protective of the gut barriers, to combat inflammation, and to resolve IBS. It regulates the gut/brain axis via the vagus nerve and stimulates hormone production in the gut. Helps reset the circadian cycles in the body. It can also reduce damage caused by long-term use of NSAIDS that can increase gastric bleeding.

- **KPV.** KPV is a powerful bioregulator in the body that treats inflammatory conditions of the gut and skin by downregulating the IL-6 and TNF-a pathways. Eases suffering for IBS, colitis, and Crohn's disease. It also has antimicrobial effects for two common pathogens in irritable bowel disease.

- **Tesofensine.** Tesofensine has shown to be incredibly helpful for weight loss by increasing serotonin, which helps with food cravings. It also improves dopamine, making you satiated faster for less overeating, and increases epinephrine, which allows you to burn fat more efficiently.

- **Semaglutide.** Clinical trials show Semaglutide to be nearly as effective as a bariatric bypass surgery or a lap band without the risks of surgery.[27] This is one of the best peptides to use for sugar cravings and lowers blood sugar.

Phase 2: CellCore Detox Supplements

Using CellCore with peptides is one of the easiest and most efficient ways to "turn up" the signaling volume in your cells.

CellCore Step 3 and Step 4 protocols are the high-quality supplements to support this phase.

CellCore Step 3 is the Whole Body Immune Support. This process will allow you to continue opening up healthy drainage pathways, including lymphatic drainage. You will also remove any remaining intestinal buildup and optimize your body's natural ability to detoxify. It includes BC-ATP (Brain Carbon ATP), CT-Minerals, LymphActiv, Para 1, Para 3, and ViRadChem Binder. What most detoxifications miss is the fact that **energy is required to eliminate interferences**, so we use BC-ATP and CT-Minerals to optimize ATP production, energy levels, and immune function.

CellCore Step 4 is the Systemic Detox in your Recharge phase. This phase promotes cleansing within and beyond the gut. It consists of BC-ATP, CT-Biotic, HM-ET Binder, KL Support, and Para 4. Para 4 helps maintain a balanced gut microbiome with herbs used traditionally to support digestive function and immunity, including celery seed, cordyceps (my favorite), holy basil, and horse tail.

While many traditional probiotics never survive the gastric secretions of your stomach, the CT-Biotic offers 11 spore-forming and non-spore-forming bacterial strains for increased digestive and detoxification support. Most of us carry around heavy metals and instead of attempting to pull them out without any additional pathways open in your body, which can create some more harm than good, we use the HM-ET (heavy metal-environmental toxin) Binder, which steps in to promote the body's natural ability to detoxify in the cells and tissues, while encouraging cellular repair throughout these processes.

Once again, to support energy production, you will continue to take BC-ATP and KL Support to optimize your mitochondrial health and energy levels, as well as support healthy drainage pathways.

Phase 2: Additional Peptides

If weight loss is a goal, you may be using these peptides:

- **Semaglutide.** A weightloss superstar. In studies, participants on average lost 15 percent of their total body weight, or approximately 30 lbs.[28] It also lowers HbA1c, protects beta cells in the pancreas for improved insulin sensitivity, decreases appetite by delaying gastric emptying, and enhances feelings of satiety. Aids in the reversal of Type 2 diabetes (not safe for Type 1 diabetics). Semaglutide improves heart rate and blood pressure, repairs damaged cardiac tissue, increases left ventricle performance, and reduces systemic vascular resistance. It aids in brain enhancement by removing beta-amyloid plaque in the brain associated with Alzheimer's disease and has been shown to improve learning and memory with increasing protection of the neurons in the brain.

- **Tesofensine.** Norepinephrine, dopamine, and serotonin reuptake inhibitors for better metabolism, impulse control, and happy weight loss. Norepinephrine stimulates fat metabolism, dopamine promotes satiety, and serotonin helps prevent overeating. It also increases Brain-Derived Neurotrophic Factor (BDNF) for learning and helps reduce depression. Studies show the effectiveness of Tesofensine on appetite control remains even after participants no longer used this peptide. Tesofensine also influences the uptake of glucose which leads to lower fat deposition.

- **AOD9604.** This peptide provides pituitary HGH activation without increasing IGF-1 or an immune response. Early studies show that this peptide tripled weight loss when compared to a placebo.[29] AOD9604 also enhances cardiac protection through the beta-3-adrenergic receptor pathways and improves cardiovascular function, endurance, and sleep.

If you have pain conditions, these peptides will be used along with regenerative medicine treatments:

- **ARA290.** Analgesic- ARA290 decreases inflammation by turning off cytokines IL-6, IL-12, and TNF-alpha which improves wound healing and tissue repair. It also reduces blood pressure, blood glucose, and autoimmunity. Effects also include stimulation of blood vessel growth, stabilization of blood pressure, calming of nerves, and pain reduction. Neuropathic pain thresholds are also improved with ARA290's impact on the small nerve fibers.

- **Thymosin Beta 4.** Thymosin Beta 4 alleviates delayed onset and post-workout muscle soreness through the VEGF pathway and activates stem cells when tissues are damaged, improving cell migration and reducing inflammation and degeneration. Additionally, it has neuroprotective properties, and its immune properties decrease beta-amyloid plaques in Alzheimer's disease and increase neuronal autophagy.

- **AOD9604.** When injected directly into a damaged joint with human tissue allographs, PRP, or other carries, AOD9604 shows improvements in cartilage structure, mobility, and improves joint function.

- **GHK-CU.** GHK is a bioregulator that cleans up genetic signaling. Research shows it mobilizes stem cells into damaged tissue.[30] It improves skin elasticity, aids in new tissue formation, increases collagen production, lowers inflammation, and is widely used for age reversal.

CHAPTER 7

DEEP DIVE: RESTORE

Look back at the previous 120 days in your Accelerate Wellness journey and identify places where you've overcome challenges, cemented new habits, and created a new baseline for yourself. Take time to recognize your accomplishments. Change is not easy, and you deserve to take pride in your efforts. Now, your 60-Day Restore phase is a reminder that you can create the life and health that you want over again!

The biggest objective in Phase 1: 60-Day Reset was to remove interferences and inflammation so that your body can detoxify and heal. Your body now has better detoxification capabilities, your stress-response axis (HPA Axis) is no longer on tilt, and you can enjoy greater levels of energy and clarity in your life.

Our second phase (Phase 2, days 61-120) concentrated primarily on putting energy back into every organ, gland, and cell in your body.

Now, in the Restore phase (days 62-180 and beyond), you'll "become young again" by discovering new ways to restore youthful energy back into everything you think and do. This phase is designed around the concept of restoring your health reserves for the healthiest future of your life. Restoring your memories of the past and reframing them to capture more meaning in your life is one of the most useful capabilities you have. You are always making up the future; why not rework your past so that you can accelerate your thinking, which in turn will accelerate your health?

This phase includes three central themes. First, anything worth doing is worth doing well. That means fixing things for good. Why put a ton of effort into something just to have the same issues crop up again? Second is no death by neglect. The Accelerate Wellness program ensures that you have restored the youth and vitality needed to make your next decade, your best decade by re-running blood labs now. This is your "report card" that analyzes how well you've progressed. The third thing that happens in this phase is if you haven't attended one of the offered retreats and received age reversal treatments, now is the time to do so!

The Restore phase focuses on building the essential foundation for longevity. Running a test called True Age will help you get an idea of how your body is aging and how to address it accordingly — for the long term — to restore the energy levels you had in your youth and infuse that energy so that it's there to last.

This phase restores better cell to cell communication through a process called cognitive enhancement, using substances called nootropics to help optimize the way that your brain works. The Restore phase also uses a device called the Sphenocath and introduces perinatal stem cell tissue in through the back of the sinuses so that it can migrate up through a nerve pathway and get into the brain effectively and safely.[31] Brain health decreases inflammation and can help with neurological conditions like Alzheimers and Parkinson's Disease.

All along the way, your health and fitness advisors are helping you adjust your exercise routines and other habits, with the idea of starting your future goals now. A big part of your future health is to be able to do enjoyable activities that are fun for you. Recreation is what we do when we're not working, and so many of us don't even have any recreational activities that we enjoy. In this phase, you will explore and identify those activities. You will also eat the right resistant starches to feed the good bacteria in your gut through guidance and mentoring on timed eating.

Finally, this phase will focus on gratitude. Every moment of progress in my life has always started with gratitude, and my favorite people to work with are those who are grateful. Gratitude helps your brain release serotonin, dopamine, and GABA, all things that are critical for restoring your health and propelling you into your future.

At the end of this phase, you'll be ready for the next program, should you desire to continue your health journey. It's called the Age Reversal Medicine program, and you can read more about that in chapter 8, so you know what's on the other side of your Accelerate Wellness journey.

> ## "This is really exciting!"
>
> I have decreased body fat and visceral fat by 13%. According to a Dexa scan, I have noticed a massive improvement in my brain health. I used to forget to eat. Now I'm eating morning meals and lunch and then having a great dinner. One of my big takeaways has been the change in testosterone without hormones. That is really exciting.
>
> *Larry, 48-year-old male, former professional athlete*

Here's what your Restore phase includes:

- **Core Daily Actions.** The daily "6 Essentials" that will support your progress during that phase. You will be asked to score yourself each day on how many of the essentials you meet.

- **Phase-Specific Peptides.** The highest quality of peptides available to assist you in bypassing many of the cellular, genetic, and mitochondrial issues that might keep you from advancing. They are specifically selected for each phase and are chosen for their safety, effectiveness, and clinical outcomes.

- **CellCore Detox Supplements.** CellCore Biosciences is the industry leader in digestive, immune, and mitochondrial health. Their customized protocols will help you restore effective cellular communication. Their products are available only through qualified health practitioners.

- **Additional Supportive Peptides.** In addition to the phase-specific peptides, we may recommend additional peptides for your unique needs.

> **A Note from Regan:** I mentioned earlier, Accelerate Wellness is a seven-month program. Each phase is 60 days, with an additional month added on as a buffer. We anticipate you will make it through the program in six months, but we've included the extra month for any delays due to travel, scheduling conflicts, etc. Consider it a bonus 30 days to allow you to continue to build your habits and fine-tune your process!

What You May Experience:

With these specific protocols, in the Restore phase, patients start to experience a sense of endurance. They notice their energy is far more consistent throughout the day, and more importantly, they also feel that they are creating a foundation that's been missing, something that allows them to be more resilient. For example, one patient, Chad, is an engineer, and he occasionally has to travel to visit project sites. He was a participant in the Accelerate Wellness program and has now moved on to the Age Reversal Medicine program.

Chad recently had to re-engineer a core component of one of the projects, and he was working day and night. He said, "In the past, I would've been incredibly exhausted. It would've taken me weeks to recover. But I just needed one day." Chad took Sunday off, and he went to work Monday as if he'd worked a normal work week. He could bounce right back, where previously he would have been down and out for an extended period of time. In addition to that resilience, Chad noticed that his brain fog was gone. He was able to stay focused on his project, even though he was working several days with very little sleep.

"I've never thought I could look this good!"

My sleep has improved by 90%. My energy's up 200%. I'm down 16 pounds, and weight loss wasn't even a goal. I've never thought I could look this good! I was a chronic sugar consumer and sugar is gone. My back feels amazing. The big thing I want to focus on next is stretching daily. I'm really enjoying the movements and exercise protocol that I'm on currently.

Pam, 52-year-old female

Core Daily Actions

Each of the three Accelerate Wellness phases includes six core daily actions — we call them your "6 Essentials" — that will support your progress during that phase. In the Restore phase, these 6 Essentials will help you look into the future, designing the life (and health) you want to live decades from now. Then you'll start building that future today!

1. **Fitness 50 at Age 100 Benchmarks.** Now that you have several months under your belt, it is time to put some fire back into your belly with the Fitness 50 concept, which was generated after a conversation with my mentor, Dan Sullivan. He always says his goal is to live to be 156, twice his current age, and he makes decisions

based on that assumption. Test yourself once per week on each of these Fitness 50 Benchmarks (see appendix) and see if you can go from Fit to Fitter to Fittest.

2. **Eating Fat Without Getting Fat.** Not only are healthy fats essential for clear cellular communication, foods like avocados, wild fish, wild game meats, offal, butter, olives, and olive oil all make food taste better, too! Without fat, you aren't as sharp mentally, you crave more sugar, and aren't satiated. Aim for 80-100 grams of healthy fats every day. Contrary to popular belief these fats *will not* make you fat, they *will not* raise cholesterol, and they *will* give your brain and heart (and taste buds) a happy boost.

3. **Resistant Starches.** When you eat, your food gets digested twice, once for you, and then again for any bacteria in your body (bacteria love to fill their belly with starches from yams, sweet potatoes, rice, plantains, green bananas, cassava, Kamut, and oats!). "Resistant" starches are those that are more difficult to digest. Instead of your body absorbing the starches in your stomach and small intestine, your bacteria can enjoy feasting on them in the large intestine. If you're looking to optimize thyroid and hormone function, don't skip out on these healthy carbs. Aim for 100- 250 grams per day.

4. **Unique Physical Abilities.** Another Dan Sullivan-ism states: "Give death no assistance!" To that end, get rid

of inflamed and degenerative areas in your body so that you can step onto your yoga mat (and into the world) with confidence. Every day, stretch, lift something heavy (60 minutes of resistance training per week lowers mortality risk by 27 percent[32]), run or move fast, and then get your 10,000 steps per day in. Get close to your maximum heart rate.

Calculate Your Maximum Heart Rate (MHR)

Determine your maximum heart rate (MHR) by subtracting your age from 220.

MHR = 220 − AGE

For instance, if you are 60, your maximum heart rate is roughly 160 beats per minute.

---

5. **Timed Eating.** Intermittent fasting is all the rage these days, namely because eating in a 12-hour or less window accelerates your body's health and reverses disease without changing much else about your habits. Insulin resistance, muscle strength, sleep, and endurance all improve in a fasting state.[33] The best way to incorporate timed eating is to simply note the time that you consume your first gram of fat, carbohydrate, or protein and give yourself 12 hours maximum before the kitchen is closed until the next morning.

For instance, if you eat at 7 am, then stop eating at 7 pm. Unless you have hypoglycemia, feel free to extend the fasting window to 14 or even 16 hours per day. Just make sure you stay hydrated and get in your protein, fats, and resistant starches during your eating window.

6. **Your Gratitude Muscle.** The most important muscle that you can build is your gratitude muscle. Researchers agree that people who feel and express more gratitude also enjoy greater levels of happiness, deeper relationships, and higher levels of accomplishment than those who don't. Try to feel grateful and angry at the same time. Did it work? When in your life were you the most grateful? How often are you working on your gratitude muscle? Restoring all things health also relates to mindsets. Before you go to bed at night, think of 3 things that you are grateful for that happened that day. Your brain will release serotonin, GABA, and dopamine which will lull you right to sleep. During your Mindset Morning, reflect on the thoughts you had before drifting off to sleep.

The 60-Day Progress Report

Score yourself each day one out of six for the number of healthy habits you participated in. Give yourself bonus points for going above and beyond light and learning a new skill, meal prep, taking peptides, and sell corn detox.

Each day, on a scale of 1 to 6, score yourself on participating in each of the 6 Essentials.

TOTAL POSSIBLE POINTS 360	YOUR SCORE:

Phase 3: Peptides

The core peptides to influence these pathways are:

- **5 Amino-1 MQ.** This peptide activates the SIRT 1 pathway for recharged AMPk and NAD+ production. It increases cellular metabolism and metabolic rate, turns off cancer pathways, stops age-related muscle wasting, and increases stem cell activation in muscles following an injury and improves contractility. It also turns off the NNMT fat storing pathway and helps shrink fat cells and deposits. It reduces risks of diabetes, atherosclerosis, kidney, liver, and cardiovascular disease by lowering cholesterol by 30 percent after 16 weeks.[34] 5 Amino-1 MQ works on the GLUT4 pathways for glucose metabolism with insulin resistance especially when combined with exercise.

- **MOTS-c.** Your MOTSc peptide triggers longevity, metabolism, and insulin sensitivity while increasing brown fat activation. It activates heat shock proteins for muscle recovery through the AMPk energy building pathway and activates type 1 collagen metabolism in bones by regulating the TGF-beta pathway for osteoblast stem cells which give way to gorgeous bone mineral density. MOTS-c lowers cardiac inflammation and improves epicardial vessel function.

- **IGF-1/LR3.** IGF-1/LR3 increases the myostatin pathway for muscle growth and recovery, and it protects muscle cells and increases proprioception. It is an exercise Memetic that activates the MyoD protein, which is triggered by exercise or damaged tissue responsible for hypertrophy. It also unlocks BDNF for neuroplasticity, prevents kidney and liver disease and even wards off dementia. IGF-1 controls inflammation and turns off autoimmunity.

- **Noopept.** Studies support Noopept's ability to enhance memory, learning, and thinking ability by increased alpha- and beta-rhythms.[35] It amplifies neurotransmission signaling between the brain cells for creativity, faster learning, and increased retention. Noopept can lead to reduced fatigue and anxiety and increased exploratory patterns in the brain. It also reduces stress and prevents cognitive decline while lowering inflammation and protecting against plaque build-up in the brain.

- **Aniracetam.** This peptide increases cognitive function and memory, improves sleep patterns, boosts energy, enhances mood via serotonin, and stimulates acetylcholine for learning. It has been shown to improve mild to moderate cognitive decline in elderly adults through improved electrical signaling in the hippocampus of the brain.[36] Aniracetam has been shown in both human and animal studies to facilitate dopamine and serotonin interactions while increasing ATP.[37]

- **Tesofensine.** Norepinephrine, dopamine, and serotonin reuptake inhibitors for better metabolism, impulse control, and happy weight loss. Norepinephrine stimulates fat metabolism, dopamine promotes satiety, and serotonin helps prevent overeating. It also increases Brain-Derived Neurotrophic Factor (BDNF) for learning, and helps reduce depression. These neurotransmitters allow you to actively engage in more meaningful work without getting burned out-every entrepreneur's dream. Researchers first looked at this peptide as a regenerative agent for Parkinson's disease but soon found participants were shedding weight and lowering blood sugar in addition to the cognitive benefits of Tesofensine.

- **Semax.** Semax restores brain tissue damage from TBIs, stroke, cognitive impairment, and dementia, and calms inflammation of the optic nerve to increase coordination. This peptide optimizes your brain's rest state for better focus, less depression, and faster learning so you feel more attentive professionally and socially and finish what you start. Semax also stimulates the expression of 24 genes that improve your brain's circulation and energy production, and it enhances brain cell activity for ideal nutritional supply for maximum productivity.

- **Dihexa.** Dihexa restores self-inflicted brain damage by improving neurogenesis, activating stem cells, and removing the toxic wasteland that has been holding your genius back. It repairs synaptic connectivity through the formation of new functional synapses that improve spatial memory, create new brain connections, and increase acetylcholine. Dihexa remits blood flow to the brain resulting in a decrease of beta-amyloid plaque and brain inflammation even if you are genetically predisposed to hearing loss, Parkinson's, or Alzheimer's.

- **Selank.** Selank calms your amygdala freak-out zone by breaking down enkephalins which express fear, anxiety, and aggressiveness. As a bonus, it gently binds on opiate receptors to blunt pain. Selank squelches your anxiety by activating 52 of the 84 genes that are responsible for GABA, making it a natural "Chill-You-Out-Benzo" that type A's dream about. Selank also might be the fastest way to get to a younger brain with a 30 percent increase in Brain Derived Neurotrophic Factor (BDNF), which improves both short- and long-term memory.

Phase 3: CellCore Detox Supplements

Your next CellCore steps in the Restore phase are the Optimize A and Optimize B protocols. The 60-Day Restore phase helps restore your ability to maintain optimal wellness and build on progress with key nutrients for cellular repair, mitochondrial health, and liver health — all of which help you create more resiliency.

Advanced **TUDCA** helps open up your liver's bile ducts to effectively metabolize fats and eliminate toxins. It helps lower cholesterol because of the digestive support and bile release. It's also a natural acid that aids the liver and regeneration.

The **ViRadChem Binder** promotes the body's natural ability to detoxify glyphosate and other toxins while supporting cellular repair. Acai, artichoke leaf, broccoli leaf, and wheatgrass provide support to the body's free radical systems. The addition of Carbon Technology also encourages increased energy production, which is essential for helping the body carry out its routine detoxification functions.

CT-iodine helps you convert TSH into T3 and T4-essential hormones for thyroid function, cognitive function, digestion, energy production, metabolism, and nervous system support. CT-Iodine is formulated with optimal ratios of iodine and iodide to support the thyroid gland and metabolism.

BC-ATP optimizes mitochondrial function by giving your body the nutrients it needs to support ATP output. You will experience improved cognitive function, mental clarity and focus, and sustained physical energy. The highly charged organic acids support metabolism and the ATP cycle in being at peak efficiency while assisting your body's natural detoxification processes. BC-ATP promotes a balanced gut microbiome, cellular renewal, and immune health and is well-tolerated by the most sensitive systems.

CT-Minerals is a liquid supplement that provides minerals derived from fulvic acid sourced from soil and decomposed plant life. These naturally occurring minerals make it easier for you to digest, absorb, and utilize nutrients for supporting cellular repair, immunity, energy production, and mental clarity.

CT-Biotic is a blend of spore-forming and non-spore-forming bacteria combined with Carbon Technology. It provides 11 bacterial strains that are essential for supporting detoxification, digestive function, and immunity. As a blend of fulvic and humic acids, Carbon Technology helps protect all bacterial strains from being destroyed or damaged by stomach acid, so that cultures are still intact by the time they reach the lower GI tract.

KL-Support activates your body's cleaning and filtering system in the kidney and liver. KL Support combines herbs and nutrients including beetroot, collinsonia (stoneroot), gynostemma, marshmallow root, milk thistle seed, NAC, and parsley leaf. Together, these support your fat metabolism, hepatic blood flow, and healthy urinary tract and bladder function, while helping the body carry out its natural detoxification processes.

Phase 3: Additional Peptides

If sexual rejuvenation is a goal, you can get the downstairs rocking with these additional peptides:

- **PT-141.** PT-141 (bremelanotide) bypasses insecurities and builds up desire by acting on the central nervous system via the melanocortin receptors. It helps erase hyperarousal disorders in women and improves sexual function in men with ED that need Viagra (sildenafil), so get your date night planned. Studies show PT-141 to have immune-protecting properties, it lowers inflammation, and it even aids in fat metabolism.

- **Gonadorelin & Kisspeptin.** Both Kisspeptin and Gonadorelin release follicle-stimulating hormone (FSH) and luteinizing hormone (LH) so you can naturally improve hormone levels while fine-tuning testosterone. They are not-to-miss peptides that not only enhance your passionate drive but also increase fertility and regulate menstrual cycle issues. They both also enhance limbic activity in the brain, increase reward-seeking behavior, and improve overall mood.

- **Melanotan II.** Melanotan II increases sexual arousal, promotes reproductive area blood flow, and binds to genes that regulate hormones. It can also improve impulse control with alcohol and eating, stabilize blood sugar, improve satiety, and aid in alertness.

CHAPTER 8

PUTTING IT ALL TOGETHER

Congratulations! You've now seen the three phases of the Accelerate Wellness program and how it all works together to create optimal levels of health, fitness, and wellbeing, quickly and most importantly, permanently. You've learned some new terms and a bit more about how your body was designed to work in a healthy manor.

Think back to the early days of your business or of a company you admire. It likely all started by creating a business plan of some detail, including products and services, growth opportunities, facilities and equipment, hiring, and more. After that plan was complete, it didn't just sit in a fancy binder on a shelf; the company's founders put the plan into action, step by step.

Remember in the introduction where you answered the question, "What would you like to experience or realize by the end of the next seven months?" That is your goal, and this book is your plan, the one you need to put into action, step by step.

Now, I have a question for you:

What's next?

Here's what I mean… It's so easy to read something and feel like you've taken action. In fact, there's a body of research that shows that your brain cannot distinguish between thinking (or reading) about something and actually doing it.[38, 39, 40]

Now that you've done the "work" of reading this book, you can feel like you've actually made changes. On one hand, that's exciting. You have some confidence now that you've taken concrete steps towards a new, healthier future. You have a glimpse of what's possible, and maybe you've even made a few small mental or habit shifts while you were reading. Fantastic!

But it's easy to let things stop there. Reading is not doing, and knowledge is not action. To create the future you want, you must have a plan and then *work the plan.* The plan is clear — the three phases of Accelerate Wellness as outlined in this book. Are you ready to move forward?

The biggest gap between knowledge and action is the lack of accountability and support. Change is hard and even more difficult when you're walking the road alone. One thing that is for sure, more than anything else, is that for you to obtain your ideal health, you can't do it alone. Many people fool themselves by thinking, "I'll just try and make a few dietary changes," or "I'm gonna start exercising more." And those things are great. But a real transformation requires healing, and healing is done with other humans. That's why a key part of the Accelerate Wellness program is your team — a group of professionals at the top of their game, assembled to ensure you stay at the top of yours. From designing a peptide protocol that addresses your needs and goals, to helping you create fast, healthy meal hacks, your team is ready, willing, and able to get you to the finish line — and beyond.

WHAT HAPPENS WHEN YOU WORK WITH EAST WEST

The first thing that happens with your wellness team is a phone call. You'll notice that from the moment you call the office, you'll feel a sense of appreciation. Every patient encounter is taken very seriously, and the people who are chosen to work with the team (and who choose to work with the team) are by far the best humans on the planet.

In that first call, you will be asked how you heard about the program. Most people come from referrals, but about ten percent find the program through the East West Health YouTube channel or podcasts, books, or through a Google search. Then it will be determined if you're a good fit for the Accelerate Wellness program.

A Special Invitation

Because you found us through this book, we've got a special invitation for you. See your personal offer in the back of this book for more information!

There is a mantra at East West Health that anything worth doing is worth doing well. The goal is to make your next decade your best, healthiest decade. To do that, it is essential to develop lifelong relationships with each other, for creating an experience that makes you want to keep coming back. That's why the very first criterion for joining the Accelerate Wellness program is looking for people who want to have a lasting relationship with their wellness team. If people are just looking for a quick fix or a transactional experience, this program may not be the right choice. Your wellness team is in it for the long term, and they hope you are, too!

The next step is taking you through a discovery day. You'll meet with a Health Ascension specialist so you know exactly what needs to be done and how the Accelerate Wellness process works. You'll be oriented to your program, so you'll learn all about the benefits. Having labs available before you meet with your doctor is important, so your Health Ascension specialist will determine what labs you need before then. You will be asked lot of questions (questions most doctors won't ask), but it's not just busywork.

TESTING, TESTING

Before you meet with a doctor, your wellness team actually takes the time to read your paperwork. That's because the second criterion is no death by neglect and no surprises. What is meant by that is any issues you have are important to know about upfront so they can be addressed, ensuring that you are getting the right tests and treatments ahead of time.

The blood tests will report your carbohydrates, fat, and protein levels. Next, will be an assessment of at your hydration, looking at minerals and vitamins. Running and reviewing your bloodwork gives you an entire lifestyle protocol and helps you massively shortcut your healing process.

In addition to your blood work and any other tests you've had recently, your digestive functions will be assessed to determine any intestinal permeability and any nutritional deficiencies, which include your DHEA levels, hormones, kidney filtration systems, lymphatic health, liver, and intestines. A marker called homocysteine will also be reviewed to see how well you methylate and detoxify in your liver. It also shows if you have a leaky blood-brain barrier, which can be deadly because it leads to chronic inflammation and accelerates the amyloid plaque buildup in the brain. That can lead to dementia and Alzheimer's.

Once all the testing is complete, the right treatment strategy will be determined, including your phases of peptides and your complete protocol. All the guesswork will be taken out of the process and made very clear and easy to follow. Your wellness team places the orders for you, and the peptides just show up every month at your house, just like Christmas! It's actually fun. Often, patients send peptide "unboxing" videos, saying, "Thanks so much for sending the peptides. I'm so excited!" Your CellCore products also come right to you in a box with very clear instructions. You just work through the CellCore steps as laid out.

"I broke old habits that were holding me back..."

Working with Andie (and everyone at East West), I learned new things and broke through old thinking habits that were holding me back. You won't get some homogenized program here, but rather a personalized approach that is specific to your individual health needs. Your health starts and ends with you, but we all need a little help and a compassionate ear.

Joey, 41-year-old male

YOUR PERSONAL ACCELERATE WELLNESS TEAM

East West Health is dedicated to fixing things for good, and that means making sure that you not only get your customized monthly supply of peptides and nutritional supplements, but also the right accountability partners and the right mentorship wellness team. This as a team approach, and a big part of the Accelerate Wellness program is accountability.

You will have check-in visits along the way with your health advisors, who are certified health coaches, because having a support partner is critical to your success. They are your touchpoint, explaining your labs, teaching you planning and meal prep, and helping with the foundational skills you'll need to get the most out of the program. You will also have a fitness advisor who will put together a nutritional program for you based on your fitness goals and put together a personalized exercise program for you. Fitness advisors know how every single muscle in your body works so that you can workout pain free, no matter what limitations you might have. Your workouts are based on your most enjoyable activities so exercise is actually fun.

You also have functional medicine providers at East West Health, many of whom have a dual degree in Eastern medicine, whom you'll be meeting with once a month. Not only do they cover labs in great detail, but they also put together customized protocols on your supplements, and they'll modify your peptides as needed. The main goal in these accelerator sessions is to help you remove any cellular interference and build up any deficiencies that are getting in the way of your health goals. Because of this unique approach and perspective, many conditions that most doctors miss are able to be identified and isolated.

A Note from Regan:
The Beauty of East and West

As you can tell from my practice name, East West Health, I believe strongly in the synergy between different modalities of science and health. At East West, we look at things much differently than most other practitioners do. To me, it's so beautiful when you can add ancient wisdom to modern scientific discoveries.

A great example is the five elements of the body in Chinese medicine. Each of your organ systems has an emotional connection. For example, if somebody is chronically fearful and they're just plagued with impending doom and anxiety, then we'll work on the kidneys because the kidneys are where we house our fear. On the flip side, the kidneys are also where we house our wisdom.

A lot of times in just purely western medicine and purely functional medicine, we dismiss the role of emotions. I think it's really powerful when you receive a much more in depth look at how things work in your body. In these functional medicine visits, the provider not only looks at the science, but also the art of medicine in understanding how your emotions, your behavior, and your lifestyle is impacting your physiology.

Finally, you become a member of the Health Accelerator community. Every Wednesday, an online group coaching class is held, offering the latest research on the newest peptides or regenerative therapies. You'll also learn some very simple techniques to make your healing process even easier, better, and faster.

If you want more, you can go to East West Health University with thousands of hours of content in the form of podcasts, videos, and books to provide a deeper dive into any topic you want to explore.

It sounds like a lot — and it is! But the most important thing to know is that this program is made incredibly straightforward and simple for you. Accelerate Wellness is a concierge service, which means anytime you have an issue or a question, you can text one of your wellness team members, and they're always available for you. It's an ABC process, and it's very easy to follow.

You can achieve long-lasting changes because you are guided every step of the way and taught what needs to happen for your body to stay healthy. Peptides are great, yet the aim is not to depend on a peptide, an herb, a supplement, and especially not on medication for your health.

THE SECRET TO YOUR SUCCESS

But the real secret to your success is that when you think that you've reached your health goals, that's when the real work begins. Why lose weight twice? Why not lose it for good? What's more valuable: temporary changes in your nutrition and fitness, only to transition back to those habits, or just making the shift for good?

It is not uncommon for people to spend hundreds of thousands of dollars over the course of a decade or more looking for answers. They go to all of these specialists in western medicine, and then they go to all the functional medicine doctors, then they go to all the naturopathic doctors, and what typically happens is that they are left on their own to figure it all out and piece together a solution.

That's the opposite of what happens in the Accelerate Wellness program, which has been a 20-year project for testing and tweaking and adjusting and refining, to know what works. By opening up the right pathways at the right time with the right treatment strategies and the right mentorship and support, you will get the results you want, and they are yours forever.

In the long run, it will save you time and an enormous amount of money because not only are you getting at the root of your health issues and making permanent changes, you're also saving yourself from costly medical conditions. The cost of a less-severe heart attack is $1 million.[41] Diabetes can cost you almost $20,000 per year.[42] Fidelity Investments estimates that the average retired couple will need to save at least $300,000 for additional medical expenses after the age of 65.[43]

The Accelerate Wellness program is one of the most cost effective ways you can start working on your health now, and you avoid these huge expenses in the future. Investing in the Accelerate Wellness program comes with this guarantee: If you don't agree that this is the best investment you've ever made in your health, your wellness team will work for free until it becomes your best investment.

Are you ready to get started? The advisors in your wellness team at East West Health are ready to assist you.

Your Turn

As you look forward to a healthier, more vibrant future, what are you most excited about?

_____

_____

_____

_____

_____

_____

What concerns do you have about achieving this future?

- Trying something new

- Sticking to the program

- Making change that will last, rather than just returning to your old habits

- Sacrificing things you love

- Additional concerns:

_____

_____

What do you think you need to help you overcome these potential obstacles?

- A proven plan

- A support system

- A real desire to change

- Additional supports:

_____

_____

CHAPTER 9

WHAT'S NEXT?

One question patients often ask is, "After I complete the seven months of the Accelerate Wellness program, am I finished? What's next?"

Many people experience such a change in their life and health that they want more. In the book, *Never Stop Healing*, I allude to the fact that health is never complete. Biology is not an exact science. It has many twists and turns, and we never want to be caught off-guard. That's why viewing your health transformation as a continuous journey is key to a lifetime of vibrancy.

A small percentage of people say they just want to move into a more maintenance phase, where they get their monthly peptides and get their blood checked regularly.

But a full 80 percent of patients say that they want more — they want to move beyond maintenance into actual longevity and age reversal.

HEALTH OPTIMIZATION AND AGE REVERSAL

For those interested in longevity, an additional program is available, allowing you to continue to make progress toward your health goals. The 12-month Health Optimization program is designed specifically as a follow-up to Accelerate Wellness. As you finish your seventh month, you have a wonderful level of momentum, and we want to capitalize on that. Through the year-long program, you will receive support in the same hands-on fashion to cement your new habits and provide you the foundation to keep moving forward with a focus on longevity, including brain health, cardiovascular function, proper blood sugar, and proper liver health digestion for continually detoxing in the body, improving your energy, and optimizing your hormones.

Here's what the program includes:

Continued Testing. For ideal results, a minimum of two blood panels, preferably three or four, over the course of the year is recommended, as well as a rerun of the digestive panel to screen for infections, ensuring that your metabolites are balanced and that there are no dysbiosis or inflammatory markers. Your metabolics for oxidative stress, mitochondrial dysfunction, and omega fatty acid imbalances will also be reviewed, in addition to making sure there are no remaining heavy metal or toxic exposures and that your methylation pathways are optimized. Your true age will be retested to see how the Accelerate Wellness program has affected your biological years.

New Protocols. This testing enables your protocol to be adjusted as necessary, including any peptides and new Cell-Core phases such as metabolic support, mycotoxin support, energy boost, or intestinal permeability.

Fitness Protocols. Through your health advising, the emphasis shifts to focus on pulling your ideal future into the present moment, continually focusing on that Fitness 50 at age 100. Most patients will be near or at their ideal weight by the end of the Accelerate Wellness program, but often there are additional goals they'd like to pursue, such as muscle-building or pursuing new activities.

A variety of other tools are implemented in the Health Optimization program, such as cold plunges, biohacking supplies, and fun gadgets like the Normatec boots, which are a lymphatic massage treatment that helps with muscle recovery, circulation, and circulation.

Continued Support. You'll continue to get the guidance you need from your expert functional medicine team. The goal is to get on top of things quickly so you can maintain and even enhance your level of health.

PEAK STATE EXPERIENCE

Patients love the monthly retreats! There's nothing else like these retreats, and you can participate at any stage of your progress. Most patients will come between month 3 and month 12 of working in the program, and then they come back once or twice a year. It's one of the most rejuvenating things that you can do for your overall health.

East West Health is not just about building a clinic, but building a community. When you come to a retreat, you meet like-minded people so you can build a community and camaraderie with others who share your goals and perspective. The beautiful facility supports this process by offering a gym, biohacking bays, acupuncture stations, a zen room, and more. You'll also get an in-depth explanation of your labs, and be taught how to interpret your own labs. You can also look forward to getting introduced to different longevity thinking tools that will assist with your mindset, because mindset is what is needed more than anything.

While you're onsite, you get to take part in some longevity treatments, from stem cell therapies to hair restoration. You'll have access to a regenerative medicine doctor doing stem cells if you choose, whether that's for the brain or the cardiovascular system. Many of the retreat participants choose to do a whole body makeover while they're onsite. Not only is it a significant cost savings, but when you're in a group setting, your body's in an amplified healing state and an even bigger transformation can occur.

Of course, while you're here, you are well-fed! The onsite chef makes amazing food, and you are taken through fitness exercises straight from the Fitness 50 protocol. You'll meet one-on-one with a fitness advisor.

Additionally, at these retreats, patients can experience peak states using psychedelics under the care of a medical doctor. These experiences take place only after significant coaching and mentoring with doctors who are certified in ketamine therapy, and with the presence of a team of therapists and other support people. One of the most exciting things about this work is the individuals who have suffered with years of anxiety, depression, or PTSD. Through this process, they have a great awakening where they start to understand what's holding them back and how to move past unresolved emotions. It can be a life-changing experience, however, it should only be undertaken with the guidance of a qualified medical professional.

ALWAYS ANOTHER STEP

The one thing that needs emphasis is that there's always the next level in your progress. If you can adopt this mindset and embrace that you're always going to be working on your health, then you can continue to make it a priority. That's what East West Health aims to help you do. Your team wants to make sure you're doing the right things at the right time and not wasting time, energy, or putting yourself at risk by playing guessing games. That way, instead of looking at this process as a grind, it becomes an enjoyable, fruitful part of your life.

APPENDIX A: PEPTIDES

HPA STRESS RESET

The peptides Selank, RG3 Synapsin, and Epitalon inspire creativity, rejuvenate sleep, and shed off years of stress.

SELANK

Dosage: Nasal spray used 1 – 3x daily as needed

HPA Axis Reset and Pain Relief - Selank works on the amygdala by breaking down enkephalins which express fear, anxiety, and aggressiveness. Those enkephalins bind on opiate receptors to blunt pain.

Serotonin, GABA, and Dopamine Regulation – Selank eases sugar and food cravings. It activates 52 of the 84 genes that are responsible for GABA, making it a natural "benzodiazepine."

Enhances Cognitive Function – a 30% increase in BDNF (short/long-term synapses) in animal studies with Selank.

Decreases Brain Inflammation - Selank has been shown to lower TNF-a, IL-6, and other pro-inflammatory cytokines by shifting T cells from Th1/TH17 to Treg in the microglia of the brain. May stop viral replication in the nasal passages.

RG3 SYNAPSIN

Dosage: Nasal spray used 1 - 3x daily as needed

RG3 (Ginsenganoids, Methylcobalamine, Nicotinamide Riboside)

HPA Axis Reset – neuroprotective, enhances memory and learning and decreases inflammation. Protects against mold exposures, chemical and emotional stressors.

Longevity – increases sirtuin pathways via NAD+ for improved cardiovascular health, DNA expression, endurance, and cognitive function.

EPITALON

Dosage: Nasal spray used 1 - 3x daily as needed

HPA Axis Reset – activates telomerase activity for longevity and interacts with CD5 for immune stem cell differentiation. Fruit flies and rats given Epitalon had a 52% decrease in mortality.

Sleep, Lipids, and Cholesterol – Epitalon balances circadian rhythms and blood lipids by activating the pCREB and the alkylamine-n-acetyltransferase pathways responsible for melatonin production.

Muscle and Skin Recovery – Epitalon targets the protein synthesis gene for better protein production and decreasing inflammation by enhancing the MMP2 pathway.

LEAN MUSCLE + ENDURANCE

Your days of muscular fitness don't have to be over just yet. Tesamorelin, CJC1295, Ipamorelin, and Sarcotropin IPA will bring back your eye of the tiger.

TESAMORELIN

Dosage: SUB Q injections 5 out of 7 days

Liver Health – proteins are well established as building blocks for muscles, and your liver is responsible for converting the proteins you eat into slabs of muscle. Tesamorelin has been shown to repair even the most damaged liver so you can re-build the frame that you want in a shorter amount of time.

Belly Fat Converter – Tesamorelin/Ipamorelin effectively turns your accumulation of mid-section overage to a defined masterpiece by working on your natural youthful growth hormone pathways.

Cardio-Brain Reset – Tesamorelin is a great way to lower non-optimal ranges of cholesterol and clean out your pipes with its inflammatory lowering and regenerative properties. This peptide also improves cognitive decline while you are putting on muscle and enjoying your favorite "Fitness 50 at age 100" challenges.

CJC1295

Dosage: SUB Q injections 5 out of 7 days

Youngevity – CJC1295 is a supercharger for muscle building and accelerates recovery by inducing delta sleep waves and resets your circadian rhythms.

Energy Factory - it's not uncommon to feel a surge of energy after injecting CJC1295. Some refer to this as a flushing feeling; I like to think of it as my get up and go is ready to go.

IPAMORELIN

Dosage: SUB Q injections 5 out of 7 days

Hunger Control – building muscle is a centerpiece of CJC1295 through the growth hormone pathway which also increases hunger. Ipamorelin tames the hunger and jumps up growth hormone by turning off somatostatin for a 7x greater release.

Overuse of Medications – Ipamorelin helps combat the side effects of glucocorticoids for pain conditions and bisphosphonates that treat osteoporosis.

SARCOTROPIN

Dosage: 4ML dose fasting

Brains with the Brawn – Sarcotropin's unique properties of GHRP's (growth hormone releasing peptide), solid amino acid stack, vitamins D3 and K2 and nootropics provides world-class, science-based age-reversal medicine that also reduces sarcopenia and keeps your blood vessels squeaky clean.

IMMUNE RESET

How to have a robust immune system at any age, even with autoimmunity and cancer therapies with ABP-7, Thymogen Alpha-1, CJC1295, Ipamorelin and KPV.

APB-7

Dosage: Daily SUB Q injections as prescribed

Short-Lived Long-Haul – ABP-7 thymulin harmonizes your immune, endocrine, and central nervous system for fast recovery from COVID and other linger-longer infections like Lyme, mold, or EBV.

From Fallout to Fall In - ABP-7 restores balance in a cytokine storm. It also calms autoimmune markers IL-6 and TNF-a for a redistribution of specialized immune cells that can now spend less energy on attacking you and more on egregious invaders and can be used to reverse the aged immune system.

THYMOGEN ALPHA 1 (TA1 FRAG)

Dosage: 1 - 2 capsules daily

Immune Reinstated – even though your T-cells decline, and your thymus gland shrinks with age, Thymogen Alpha-1 (a thymosin alpha-1 frag) brings them back to life no matter what chronic infection is in the way.

Remodulation – fungal, viral, and bacterial infections can be subtle and devastating to your health, thymogen alpha-1 activates dendritic cells to release antigens that allow your immune system to ward off impending invaders without disturbing your delicate ecosystem.

Odd Cells Out – Thymogen Alpha 1 is part of your insurance policy against cancer cells by increasing CD-4 and CD-8 cells to stop tumor growth and can be used as adjunctive therapy with chemo and radiation.

CJC1295 / IPAMORELIN

Dosage: SUB Q injections 5 days on, 2 days off

Intelligent Immunity – declining growth hormone leads to an involuted thymus gland and immunity decline. CJC1295 recharges your immune cells intelligence by providing an increase of natural growth hormone. The Ipamorelin is the supercharger that yields 7x greater of a release.

KPV

Dosage: Daily SUB Q injections, or oral ingestion as prescribed

Regulate It – KPV is a small peptide chain of 3 amino acids that works like the conductor of your genetic orchestra and turns on genetic expression with just the right pitch while silencing those off-tune so that your innate and adaptive immune response aligns to protect you when you need it most.

Healing Energy – KPV works on a pathway in Chinese Medicine known as the Wei Qi, or the Protective Force, which is an invisible energy field circulating on the outside of your skin. I think that the Wei Qi pathway is the alpha-melanocyte-stimulating hormone, which modulates skin pigmentation and immunity.

Fever Reduction – KPV cools the inflammatory fire in feverish conditions via the MSHalpha pathways.

YOUR BEST WEIGHT

When it comes to looking and feeling your best, Semaglutide, Tesofinsine, and AOD9604 are your go-to fat melting peptides.

SEMAGLUTIDE (GLP-1)

Dosage: Weekly SUB Q injections as prescribed

Weight Loss Superstar – study participants on average lost 15% of their total body weight or approximately 30 pounds.

Blood Sugar/Diabetes – lowers HbA1c, protects beta cells in the pancreas for improved insulin sensitivity, decreases appetite by delaying gastric emptying, and enhances feelings of satiety. Aids in reversal of Type 2 diabetes but not safe for Type 1 diabetics.

Cardio-protective – Semaglutide improves heart rate and blood pressure. Repairs damaged cardiac tissue following an event. Increases left ventricle performance and reduces systemic vascular resistance.

Brain Enhancement – removes beta-amyloid plaque in the brain associated with Alzheimer's disease, and has been shown to improve learning and memory with increased protection of the neurons in the brain.

TESOFENSINE

Dosage: 1 capsule in the morning

Happy Weight Loss – norepinephrine, dopamine, and serotonin reuptake inhibitors for better metabolism, impulse control, and happy weight loss. Norepinephrine stimulates fat metabolism, dopamine promotes satiety, and serotonin helps prevent overeating. Increases BDNF for learning and reduces depression.

Lose Weight for Good – the effectiveness of Tesofensine on appetite control remains even after participants no longer used this peptide, leading to favorable long-term eating patterns, not dependent on willpower.

Insulin Resistance – Tesofensine influences the uptake of glucose which leads to lower fat deposition.

AOD9604

Dosage: SUB Q injections or apply directly to stubborn adipose deposits.

Lose Weight, Feel Young – Pituitary HGH activation without increasing IGF-1 or an immune response. Early studies show that this peptide tripled weight loss when compared to a placebo in 300 obese individuals.

Healthy Heart - AOD9604 enhances cardiac protection through the beta-3-adrenergic receptor pathways. Improves cardiovascular function, endurance, and sleep.

Pain-Free Joints – research shows that AOD9604 injected directly into joints may aid in the regeneration of osteoarthritic joints and may help improve stem cell proliferation when used with perinatal tissue.

GUT RECHARGE

Fix your gut for good with the most potent peptides available, LL37, BPC157, KPV, and VIP, to remove, repair, and restore harmony to your invaluable energy generator - the gut.

LL37

Dosage: LL37 is naturally secreted in humans only as a response to infections and is one of the body's most advanced anti-microbial, anti-viral, anti-bacterial, anti-fungal, and antiinflammatory peptides. It might be the most promising replacement for antibiotics because of its ability to select pathogenic from friendly microbes.

Leaky Gut – LL37 downregulates TL4 and increases IL-18 to decrease inflammation, repairs leaky gut by binding on lipopolysaccharides (LPS) to stop bacterial translocation and repairs compromised barriers.

SIBO and Biofilms – Useful for IBS or any acute or chronic infections. Breaks down biofilms in SIBO, mold, and Lyme disease, and corrects inflammatory conditions of the intestines.

BPC-157

Dosage: Daily SUB Q injections as prescribed

BPC157 (body protective complex) was first isolated from human gastric juices and has been shown to be protective of gut barriers, combats inflammation, and resolves IBS.

Heals Barriers – BPC157 stimulates nitric oxide for new vessel growth. It regulates the gut/brain axis via the vagus nerve and stimulates hormone production in the gut. Helps reset the circadian cycles in the body.

Overuse of Medication – the body protective complex reduces damage caused by long-term use of NSAIDS that increase gastric bleeding.

KPV

Dosage: Daily oral, topical, or SUB Q injections as prescribed

KPV is a powerful bioregulator in the body that treats inflammatory conditions of the gut and skin by downregulating the IL-6 and TNF-a pathways. Eases suffering from IBS, colitis, and Crohn's disease.

Infections – KPV works on the alpha-MSH pathway, and its antimicrobial effects have been demonstrated on S. aureus and C. Albicans, two common pathogens in irritable bowel disease.

VIP

Dosage: Daily nasal spray as prescribed

Vasoactive Intestinal peptide relaxes the smooth muscle in the gut, lowers blood pressure, and aids the immune function with mold and Lyme exposure. Balances the parasympathetic nervous system.

INNER GENIUS

What if you could think, learn, and act on the things that matter most to you? Noopept, Aniracetam, and Tesofensine are designed to get you there on time, every time - with a smile.

NOOPEPT

Dosage: Take 1 AM capsule 3 to 4 x per week

Supercharged Brain – studies support Noopept's ability to enhance memory, learning, and thinking ability by increased alpha- and beta-rhythms.

Electric Brain – Noopept amplifies neurotransmission signaling between the brain cells for creativity, faster learning, and increased retention.

Faster Focus – reduced fatigue, anxiety, and increased exploratory patterns in the brain. Reduces stress and prevents cognitive decline. Lowers inflammation and protects against plaque build-up in the brain.

ANIRACETAM

Dosage: Take 1 AM capsule 3 - 4 times per week w/ choline

Creative Output – increases cognitive function and memory, and improves sleep patterns. Aniracetam boosts energy, enhances mood via serotonin, and stimulates acetylcholine for learning.

Neuro-Plasticity – aniracetam improved mild to moderate cognitive decline in elderly adults through improved electrical signaling in the hippocampus of the brain.

Happy Energy – everyone is happier with an optimized brain, and aniracetam has been shown in both human and animal studies to facilitate dopamine and serotonin interactions while increasing ATP.

TESOFENSINE

Dosage: Take 1 AM capsule daily as prescribed

Emotionally Fit – Tesofensine enhances norepinephrine, dopamine, and serotonin to provide you with focused serenity while also increasing BDNF for learning and cognitive function. These neurotransmitters allow you to actively engage in more meaningful work without getting burned out-every entrepreneur's dream.

Your Brain and 6-Pack Optimized – Tesofensine activates norepinephrine to stimulate fat metabolism, dopamine to promote satiety, and serotonin so that you ditch the food coma. Researchers first looked at this peptide as a regenerative agent for Parkinson's disease but soon found out that their participants were shedding weight and lowering blood sugar while reaping the cognitive benefits of Tesofensine.

ENERGY + MITO RESTORE

Restoring energy has never been easier with 5 amino-1-MQ, MOTSc, and IGF-1. Feel faster on your feet, summit mountains in less time, and activate your metabolism.

5 AMINO 1 MQ

Dosage: 1 Pill per week for 1 week / two pills per week for two weeks/ 3 pills until gone

Energy and Longevity Recharge – activates the SIRT 1 pathway for recharged AMPk and NAD+ production. Increases cellular metabolism and metabolic rate. Turns off cancer pathways for greater longevity.

Athleticism – stops age-related muscle wasting, increases stem cell activation in muscles following an injury, and improves contractility by 70%.

Weight loss – 5-amino-1-MQ turns off the NNMT fat-storing pathway and helps shrink fat cells and deposits. It reduces risks of diabetes, atherosclerosis, kidney, liver, and cardiovascular disease by lowering cholesterol by 30% after 16 weeks.

Insulin Sensitivity – 5-amino-1-MQ works on the GLUT4 pathways for glucose metabolism with insulin resistance especially when combined with exercise.

IGF-1 / LR3

Dosage: SUB Q injections 5 of 7 days

Muscle Recharge – IGF-1/LR3 increases the myostatin pathway for muscle growth and recovery. It protects muscle cells and increases proprioception. IGF-1/LR3 is an exercise Memetic that activates the MyoD protein, which is triggered by exercise or damaged tissue responsible for hypertrophy.

Nootropic and Longevity – IGF1 is the key that unlocks BDNF for neuroplasticity. IGF-1 prevents kidney and liver disease and even wards off dementia. IGF-1 controls inflammation and turns off autoimmunity.

MOTS-C

Dosage: 1 ML SUB Q injections or as prescribed

10x Exercise Capacity – your MOTS-c peptide triggers longevity, metabolism, and insulin sensitivity while increasing brown fat activation. MOTS-c activates heat shock proteins for muscle recovery through the AMPk energy-building pathway.

Goodbye Osteoporosis – MOTS-c activates type 1 collagen metabolism in bones by regulating the TGF-beta pathway for osteoblast stem cells which give way to gorgeous bone mineral density.

Age Reversal Medicine – MOTS-c is more expressed in Japanese populations that live longer. It has also been shown that patients with heart disease have lower levels of MOTS-c and more endothelial cell damage. MOTS-c lowers cardiac inflammation and improves epicardial vessel function.

PAIN + REGENERATION

Peptides to help you restore, repair, regenerate, and feel your absolute best.

ARA290

Dosage: SUB Q injection daily as prescribed

Analgesic – ARA290 decreases inflammation by turning off cytokines IL-6, IL-12, and TNF-alpha which improves wound healing and tissue repair. Reduces blood pressure, blood glucose, and autoimmunity.

Repairs – ARA290 stimulates blood vessel growth, stabilizes blood pressure, calms nerves, and reduces pain.

Nerve Pain – neuropathic pain thresholds are improved with ARA290's impact on the small nerve fibers.

BPC157

Dosage: SUB Q injection daily as prescribed

Heals Damaged Areas – BPC157 stimulates nitric oxide for new vessel growth and increases fibroblasts for tendon repair in a more effective way than most other therapies.

Overuse of Medication – the body protective complex reduces damage caused by long-term use of NSAIDS that increase gastric bleeding. BPC157 is effective against cortisone injection overuse.

THYMOSIN BETA 4

Dosage: Daily oral, topical, or SUB Q injections as prescribed

Muscle Soreness – alleviates delayed onset and post-workout muscle soreness through the VEGF pathway.

Stem Cell Recruitment – the Thymosin Beta 4 gene activates stem cells when tissues are damaged which improves cell migration, inflammation, and degeneration.

Brain Health – Thymosin Beta 4 has neuroprotective properties and its immune properties decrease beta-amyloid plaques in Alzheimer's disease and increase neuronal autophagy.

AOD9604

Dosage: Applied topically on injured area, or SUB Q injection

Joint Pain – AOD9604 when injected directly into a damaged joint with human tissue allografts, PRP, or other carriers, shows improvements in cartilage structure, and mobility, and improves joint function.

GHK-CU

Dosage: Applied topically on injured area, or SUB Q injection

Genetic Sweeping – GHK is a bioregulator that cleans up genetic signaling, and research shows it mobilizes stem cells into damaged tissue. Improves skin elasticity and aids in new tissue formation.

Collagen – GHK increases collagen production, lowers inflammation, and is widely used for age reversal.

COGNITIVE RECLAMATION

Take it or leave it. Your most impressive traits, skills, and thoughts reside right inside your cranium. Semax, DIHEXA, and Selank keep the engine purring while you reclaim what was lost.

SEMAX

Dosage: Morning nasal spray daily or as prescribed

BDNF – Semax restores brain tissue damage from TBIs, stroke, cognitive impairment, and dementia, and calms inflammation of the optic nerve so that you make your coordination and inner athlete great again.

Serotonin and Dopamine Reset – Semax optimizes your brain's rest state for better focus, less depression, and faster learning so that you feel more attentive professionally and socially, and finish what you start.

Smart Genes – Semax stimulates the expression of 24 genes that improve your brain's circulation and energy production and enhance brain cell activity for an ideal nutritional supply for maximum productivity.

DIHEXA

Dosage: Take 1 pill daily or apply directly on carotid artery

Protect Your Brain – DIHEXA restores self-inflicted brain damage by improving neurogenesis, activating stem cells, and removal of the toxic wasteland that has been holding your genius back.

Boosts Your Memory (for good) – DIHEXA repairs synaptic connectivity through the formation of new functional synapses that improve spatial memory and new brain connections, and increases acetylcholine.

Hearing Loss Alzheimer's and Parkinson's Protection – DIHEXA remits blood flow to the brain resulting in a decrease of beta-amyloid plaque and brain inflammation, even if you are genetically predisposed.

SELANK

Dosage: Morning nasal spray daily or as prescribed.

Good Mood – Selank calms your amygdala freak-out zone, by breaking down enkephalins that express fear, anxiety, and aggressiveness… as a bonus, it gently binds on opiate receptors to blunt pain.

GABA-tized – Selank's shortcut to quelch your anxiety occurs by activating 52 of the 84 genes that are responsible for GABA, making it a natural "Chill-You-Out-Benzo" that type A's dream about.

Youthful Spark – imagine having your brain's youthful spark restored. Selank might be the fastest way to get there with a 30% increase in BDNF which improves both short/long-term memory.

Brain on Fire to Fire Brain – Selank has been shown to lower TNF-a, IL-6, and other pro-inflammatory cytokines by shifting T cells from Th1/TH17 to Treg which are also fancy molecules that prevent infections.

SEXUAL REJUVENATION

Get the downstairs rocking with PT-141, Kisspectin, and Melanotan 2. Forget about worrisome moments of unfulfilled passion and enjoy your long-awaited love adventures.

PT-141

Dosage: Nasal spray or SUB Q injection 30 minutes before sexy times

Get That Sexual Feeling – PT-141 (bremelanotide) bypasses insecurities and builds up desire by acting on the central nervous system via the melanocortin receptors.

Female and Male Enjoyment – PT-141 helps erase hyper-arousal disorders in women and even improved sexual function in men with ED better than Viagra (sildenafil), so get your date night planned.

Studies show PT-141 to have immune-protecting properties, lowers inflammation, and it even aids in fat metabolism.

GONADORELIN + KISSPECTIN

Dosage: SUB Q injection 2-7 x per week

Vitality – both Kisspectin and Gonadorelin releases FSH and LH so that you can naturally improve hormone levels while fine-tuning testosterone specifically.

Fertility Quotient – Gonadorelin and Kisspectin are not to miss peptides that have robust properties to not only enhance your passionate drive but it also increases fertility and regulates menstrual irregularities.

Brings on the Good Moods – no one wants to make love with a grump. Both Kisspectin and Gonadorelin foster enhanced limbic activity in the brain, increased reward-seeking behavior, and improved overall mood.

MELANOTAN 2

Dosage: SUB Q injections 2 - 7 x per week

Arousal Activator – beyond getting darker skin pigmentation, Melanotan 2 increases sexual arousal, promotes reproductive area blood flow, and binds to genes that regulate hormones.

Stimulation with Impulse Control – Melanotan 2 increases sexual arousal while also improving impulse control with alcohol and eating.

Bonus Territory – Melanotan 2 helps stabilize blood sugar, improves satiety, and also aids in alertness.

APPENDIX B: FITNESS 50 BENCHMARKS

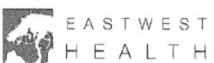

EASTWEST
HEALTH

Your Fitness 50 Benchmarks

FIT			FITTER	
Push Ups: 50 Seconds	15		Push Ups: 50 Seconds	25
Plank Hold	1 Minute		Plank Hold	2 Minute
Grip Test: Dead hang	30 Seconds		Grip Test: Dead hang	60 Seconds
Squats: 50 Seconds	20		Squats: 50 Seconds	35
Wall Squat Hold	30 Seconds		Wall Squat Hold	60 Seconds
Lunges: 50 Seconds	20		Lunges: 50 Seconds	35
Sit-To-Stand: 50 Seconds	3		Sit-To-Stand: 50 Seconds	5
Sit-To-Rise: No Hands	2		Sit-To-Rise: No Hands	1
Single Leg Balance: 50 Seconds	20		Single Leg Balance: 50 Seconds	35
1-Mile Walk/Run/Elliptical	12 Minutes		1-Mile Walk/Run/Elliptical	10 Minutes
50 Burpees	4 Minutes		50 Burpees	3 Minutes
ACHIEVED			ACHIEVED	

KEY INSIGHTS

FITNESS 50 AT AGE 100 BENCHMARK ASCENSION
Dan Sullivan and Regan Archibald Lifetime Extender Collaboration

For most of us, living to 100 won't be an issue. What will be of concern, though, is our quality of life when we get there. Imagine having the fitness level of the healthiest 50-year-old at the age of 100. It is possible — if you start now. Your future self will appreciate the time you spend taking care of your health, and the Fitness 50 Benchmarks are a simplified way to increase longevity. The purpose is to have a baseline fitness threshold that you can enjoy when you are 100.

Each of the Fitness 50 Benchmarks can be viewed as diagnostic predictors of diseases caused by aging and are early indicators for all-cause mortality. They are also the easiest way to measure progress towards your goal. No blood draws, stool tests, or DNA swabs are needed.

The three levels are Fit, Fitter, and Fittest. Use them as motivation to make improvements no matter what your age or fitness level. I suggest working on each of the 11 benchmarks in one session once a week, but feel free to perform some of the benchmarks in groups, or test them individually.

Successfully go to Fit to Fitter to Fittest in each category

FITTEST	
Push Ups: 50 Seconds	40
Plank Hold	3 Minute
Grip Test: Dead hang	90 Seconds
Squats: 50 Seconds	50
Wall Squat Hold	90 Seconds
Lunges: 50 Seconds	50
Sit-To-Stand: 50 Seconds	7
Sit-To-Rise: No Hands	0
Single Leg Balance: 50 Seconds	50
1-Mile Walk/Run/Elliptical	8 Minutes
50 Burpees	2 Minutes
ACHIEVED	

Push Ups = being able to perform 40 push-ups (with modifications if necessary) can indicate a substantially reduced risk of stroke and heart disease,[44] and is associated with increased strength and improved growth hormone. *Cardiovascular Health and Strength*

Plank Hold = improves posture, strengthens the core, and increases flexibility and endurance. Planks increase the basal metabolic rate, decrease fat percentage, and improve immunocyte counts.[45] *Metabolism, Flexibility, Strength, Endurance, and Immune Function*

Grip strength = increase in strength reduces blood pressure and risk of stroke. Improves testosterone, growth hormone, and signals muscle readiness for the entire body through the brain and can be a stand in measurement for full body strength and muscle mass.[46] *Cardiovascular Health and Strength*

Wall Squat Hold = enhances lower body stability and strength while reducing resting blood pressure and improving lumbar stability. *Balance, Alignment, Cardiovascular Health, Strength*

Lunges = benefits the posterior muscles (hamstrings, glutes, and low back) better than other movements. Corrects instability and improves balance. *Strength, Balance, and Alignment*

Sit to Stand = core strength, endurance, and balance and is a predictor of mortality.[47] *Strength, Balance, Endurance*

Sit to Rise = musculoskeletal fitness predictor for longevity, balance, and coordination. *Strength, Balance, and Coordination*

Single Leg Balance = related to decrease occurrence of strokes and cognitive decline,[48] improves cerebral circulation and vascular health. *Flexibility, Balance, and Cardiovascular Health*

1-Mile Run/Elliptical/Rowing/Swimming = improves cardiovascular function, decreases chances of stroke, improves endurance and strength. Increases cognitive function and fitness. Rowing, swimming, and the elliptical are all alternatives to running. Feel free to test yourself on any endurance related activity for 8-12 minutes to see how you fare. *Endurance, Cardiovascular Fitness, and Brain Health*

Burpees = increase blood flow, lowers blood pressure, improves strength, coordination, and endurance. Stimulates fat burning and metabolism and lowers risk of all-cause mortality.[49] *Endurance, Fitness, Strength, and Cardiovascular Health*

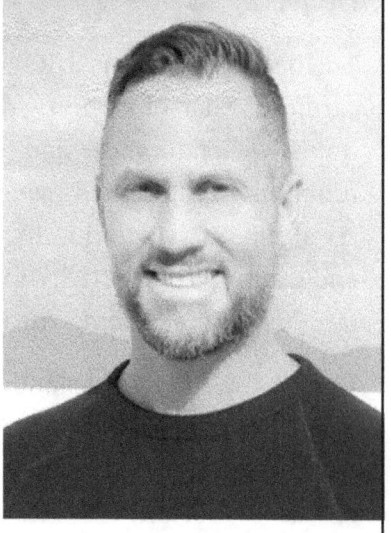

ABOUT REGAN ARCHIBALD

Regan Archibald, Lac, FMP, is one of the nation's leading peptide specialists and is the founder of East West Health, the award-winning clinic he founded in 2004. East West Health is the first Medically Managed Peptide Program that includes the use of acupuncture and herbs, regenerative medicine, and functional medicine. He is the founder of Go Wellness, the creator of the Peptide Mastery Course, and a member of the International Peptide Society.

As a peptide expert, Licensed Acupuncturist, and Functional Medicine Practitioner, Regan brings innovation and cutting-edge options to those looking to recover from pain, to balance hormones, to increase performance, or to optimize their health. You can hear more about his unique approach to health via his podcast, Never Stop Healing.

If not teaching, writing, or working with patients in-office or virtually, you will find Regan in the Wasatch mountains with his wife Jessica and his kids, Zoe, Dominic, and Jonah. He loves to ski, snowboard, mountain bike, take ice baths, and bio-hack, and is passionate about bringing art back into the practice of medicine.

Find out more at ThePeptideExpert.com.

ENDNOTES

1 Health and Retirement Study, 2017 Spring Life History Mail Survey (LHMS) public use dataset. Produced and distributed by the University of Michigan with funding from the National Institute on Aging (grant number NIA U01AG009740). Ann Arbor, MI, (2021).

2 Li, Y., Pan, A., Wang, D. D., Liu, X., Dhana, K., Franco, O. H., Kaptoge, S., Angelantonio, E. D., Stampfer, M., Willett, W. C., & Hu, F. B. (2018, April 30). Impact of healthy lifestyle factors on life expectancies in the US population. Circulation. Retrieved November 9, 2022, from https://www.ahajournals.org/doi/10.1161/CIRCULATIONA-HA.117.032047

3 Fang, M., Wang, D., Coresh, J., & Selvin, E. (2022, July 11). Undiagnosed diabetes in U.S. adults: Prevalence and trends. American Diabetes Association. Retrieved October 26, 2022, from https://diabetesjournals.org/care/article/45/9/1994/147216/Undiagnosed-Diabetes-in-U-S-Adults-Prevalence-and-trends

4 What happens during a heart attack (infographic). What Happens During a Heart Attack - UnityPoint Health. (n.d.). Retrieved October 27, 2022, from https://www.unitypoint.org/livewell/article.aspx?id=05a80ce6-a1e4-4ad4-b7c8-48645d2ba703

5 Kubala, J. (2020, January 20). Can you overdose on vitamins? Healthline. Retrieved October 28, 2022, from https://www.healthline.com/nutrition/can-you-overdose-on-vitamins#:~:text=Given%20that%20fat%2Dsoluble%20vitamins,harmful%20side%20effects%20(%205%20)

6 Commissioner, O. (n.d.). Mixing medications and dietary supplements can endanger your health. U.S. Food and Drug Ad-

ministration. Retrieved October 28, 2022, from https://www.fda. gov/consumers/consumer-updates/mixing-medications-and-dietary-supplements-can-endanger-your-health#:~:text=Combining%20dietary%20supplements%20and%20medications,John's%20wort%2C%20an%20herbal%20supplement.

7   Wang, L., Wang, N., Zhang, W., Cheng, X., Yan, Z., Shao, G., Wang, X., Wang, R., & Fu, C. (2022, February 14). Therapeutic peptides: Current applications and Future Directions. Nature News. Retrieved October 28, 2022, from https://www.nature.com/articles/s41392-022-00904-4#:~:text=Since%20the%20synthesis%20of%20the,hottest%20topics%20in%20pharmaceutical%20research.

8   An interview with prof. Khavinson. Peptides Store. (2011). Retrieved December 12, 2022, from https://www.peptidesstore.com/blogs/articles/15207153-an-interview-with-prof-khavinson

9   staff, S. X. (2018, June 4). The long and the short of DNA replication. Phys.org. Retrieved October 28, 2022, from https://phys.org/news/2018-06-short-dna-replication.html

10   U.S. National Library of Medicine. (n.d.). Hormones | endocrine glands. MedlinePlus. Retrieved October 28, 2022, from https://medlineplus.gov/hormones.html

11   Walter, K. (2021, February 4). Nearly 40% of adults suffer from a functional gastrointestinal disorder. HCPLive. Retrieved October 28, 2022, from https://www.hcplive.com/view/40-percent-adults-functional-gastrointestinal-disorder

12   Powell, M. (2018, March 26). At the heart of a vast doping network, an alias. The New York Times. Retrieved October 28, 2022,

from https://www.nytimes.com/2018/03/26/sports/doping-thom-as-mann-peptides.html

13 Naviaux R. K. (2014). Metabolic features of the cell danger response. Mitochondrion, 16, 7–17. https://doi.org/10.1016/j.mito.2013.08.006

14 U.S. National Library of Medicine. (n.d.). Hormones | endocrine glands. MedlinePlus. Retrieved October 28, 2022, from https://medlineplus.gov/hormones.html

15 Albert Sanchez, J. L. Reeser, H. S. Lau, P. Y. Yahiku, R. E. Willard, P. J. McMillan, S. Y. Cho, A. R. Magie, U. D. Register, Role of sugars in human neutrophilic phagocytosis, The American Journal of Clinical Nutrition, Volume 26, Issue 11, November 1973, Pages 1180–1184, https://doi.org/10.1093/ajcn/26.11.1180

16 U.S. National Library of Medicine. (n.d.). Hypothalamus: Medlineplus medical encyclopedia. MedlinePlus. Retrieved November 2, 2022, from https://medlineplus.gov/ency/article/002380.htm#:~:text=The%20hypothalamus%20is%20an%20area,Hunger

17 About the pituitary gland. Barrow Neurological Institute. (2022, June 28). Retrieved November 2, 2022, from https://www.barrowneuro.org/resource/about-the-pituitary-gland/

18 Adrenal glands. Adrenal Glands | Johns Hopkins Medicine. (2021, August 8). Retrieved November 2, 2022, from https://www.hopkinsmedicine.org/health/conditions-and-diseases/adrenal-glands

19 Sheng, J. A., Bales, N. J., Myers, S. A., Bautista, A. I., Roueinfar, M., Hale, T. M., & Handa, R. J. (1AD, January 1). The hypothalamic-pituitary-adrenal axis: Development, programming actions of hormones, and maternal-fetal interactions. Frontiers. Retrieved No-

vember 2, 2022, from https://www.frontiersin.org/articles/10.3389/fnbeh.2020.601939/full#:~:text=A%20major%20component%20of%20the,autonomic%20nervous%20system%20(ANS)

20 Mayo Foundation for Medical Education and Research. (2021, November 13). Human growth hormone (HGH): Does it slow aging? Mayo Clinic. Retrieved November 2, 2022, from https://www.mayoclinic.org/healthy-lifestyle/healthy-aging/in-depth/growth-hormone/art-20045735

21 Sarma, S, Palcu, P. Weight loss between glucagon-like peptide-1 receptor agonists and bariatric surgery in adults with obesity: A systematic review and meta-analysis. Obesity (Silver Spring). 2022; 30(11): 2111- 2121. doi:10.1002/oby.23563

22 MediLexicon International. (n.d.). Flow state: Definition, examples, and how to achieve it. Medical News Today. Retrieved November 4, 2022, from https://www.medicalnewstoday.com/articles/flow-state

23 van der Linden, D., Tops, M., & Bakker, A. B. (1AD, January 1). The neuroscience of the flow state: Involvement of the locus coeruleus norepinephrine system. Frontiers. Retrieved November 4, 2022, from https://www.frontiersin.org/articles/10.3389/fpsyg.2021.645498/full

24 ScienceDaily. (2022, July 25). New Study finds lowest risk of death was among adults who exercised 150-600 minutes/week. ScienceDaily. Retrieved November 4, 2022, from https://www.sciencedaily.com/releases/2022/07/220725105618.htm

25 Starrett, J. (2021, May 19). Why everyone should be eating organ meats. The Ready State. Retrieved November 4, 2022, from https://

thereadystate.com/blogs/why-everyone-should-be-eating-or-gan-meats/#:~:text=Studies%20show%20adding%20organ%20meats,increases%20the%20need%20for%20iron.

26 Marcelo Campos, M. D. (2021, November 16). Leaky gut: What is it, and what does it mean for you? Harvard Health. Retrieved November 4, 2022, from https://www.health.harvard.edu/blog/leaky-gut-what-is-it-and-what-does-it-mean-for-you-2017092212451

27 Sarma, S, Palcu, P. Weight loss between glucagon-like peptide-1 receptor agonists and bariatric surgery in adults with obesity: A systematic review and meta-analysis. Obesity (Silver Spring). 2022; 30(11): 2111- 2121. doi:10.1002/oby.23563

28 Wilding, J. P. H., Rosen, C. J., Ingelfinger, J. R., Devos, D., Suarez, E. A., Epstein, J. N., Komakech, D., Cowger, T. L., Chalkias, S., & Ssenkumba, B. (2021, March 18). Once-weekly semaglutide in adults with overweight or obesity: Nejm. New England Journal of Medicine. Retrieved December 2, 2022, from https://www.nejm.org/doi/full/10.1056/NEJMoa2032183

29 Obesity drug codenamed AOD9604 highly successful in trials. News. (2019, June 19). Retrieved December 2, 2022, from https://www.news-medical.net/news/2004/12/16/6878.aspx

30 Pickart, L., Vasquez-Soltero, J. M., & Margolina, A. (2015, July 7). GHK peptide as a natural modulator of multiple cellular pathways in skin regeneration. BioMed research international. Retrieved December 2, 2022, from https://www.ncbi.nlm.nih.gov/pmc/articles/PMC4508379/

31 The Sphenocath can be one of the most phenomenal treatments

ever. I actually wrote a book about this entire process called Brain Rejuvenation, and I recommend you check it out. This treatment has helped hundreds of our patients who have neurological conditions like Parkinson's and Alzheimer's.

32 Shailendra P; Baldock KL; Li LSK; Bennie JA; Boyle T; (n.d.). Resistance training and mortality risk: A systematic review and meta-analysis. American journal of preventive medicine. Retrieved November 25, 2022, from https://pubmed.ncbi.nlm.nih. gov/35599175/#:~:text=A%20dose%2Dresponse%20meta%2Danalysis,CI%3D0.64%2C%200.86)

33 Panda, S. (2018). The circadian code: Lose weight, supercharge your energy, and Transform Your Health from morning to midnight. Rodale.

34 Neelakantana, H., Vancea, V., Wetzelbc, M. D., Wangd, H.-Y. L., McHardyd, S. F., Finnertybc, C. C., Hommele, J. D., & Watowicha, S. J. (2017, November 15). Selective and membrane-permeable small molecule inhibitors of nicotinamide N-methyltransferase reverse high fat diet-induced obesity in mice. Biochemical Pharmacology. Retrieved December 2, 2022, from https://www.sciencedirect.com/ science/article/abs/pii/S0006295217306718?via%3Dihub

35 Patel, K. (2022, November 17). N-phenylacetyl-L-prolylglycine ethyl ester. Examine. Retrieved December 2, 2022, from https://examine. com/supplements/noopept/research/

36 Koliaki, C. C., Messini, C., & Tsolaki, M. (2012, April 18). Clinical efficacy of aniracetam, either as monotherapy or combined with cholinesterase inhibitors, in patients with Cognitive Impairment: A Comparative Open Study. CNS neuroscience & therapeutics. Re-

trieved December 2, 2022, from https://www.ncbi.nlm.nih.gov/pmc/articles/PMC6493642/

37 Shirane, M., & Nakamura, K. (2001, October 19). Aniracetam enhances cortical dopamine and serotonin release via cholinergic and glutamatergic mechanisms in Shrsp. Brain research. Retrieved December 2, 2022, from https://pubmed.ncbi.nlm.nih.gov/11597608/

38 https://exploringyourmind.com/your-brain-when-you-read-what-happens/

39 Pascual-Leone A;Nguyet D;Cohen LG;Brasil-Neto JP;Cammarota A;Hallett M; (n.d.). Modulation of muscle responses evoked by transcranial magnetic stimulation during the acquisition of New Fine Motor Skills. Journal of neurophysiology. Retrieved November 27, 2022, from https://pubmed.ncbi.nlm.nih.gov/7500130/

40 Copyright © 2006-2022 OEDb.org, a Red Ventures Company. (2016, March 31). Your brain on books: 10 ways reading affects psyche. OEDB.org. Retrieved November 27, 2022, from https://oedb.org/ilibrarian/your-brain-on-books-10-things-that-happen-to-our-minds-when-we-read/#:~:text=When%20we%20read%2C%20the%20brain,same%20neurological%20regions%20are%20stimulated

41 Vernon, S. (2010, April 23). How much would a heart attack cost you? CBS News. Retrieved December 2, 2022, from https://www.cbsnews.com/news/how-much-would-a-heart-attack-cost-you/

42 The cost of diabetes. The Cost of Diabetes | ADA. (2017). Retrieved December 2, 2022, from https://diabetes.org/about-us/statistics/cost-diabetes#:~:text=People%20with%20diagnosed%20diabetes%20incur,in%20the%20absence%20of%20diabetes

43 Fidelity releases 2022 retiree health care cost estimate: 65-year-

old couple retiring today will need an average of $315,000 for medical expenses. Business Wire. (2022, May 16). Retrieved December 2, 2022, from https://www.businesswire.com/news/home/20220516005224/en/Fidelity-Releases-2022-Retiree-Health-Care-Cost-Estimate-65-Year-Old-Couple-Retiring-Today-Will-Need-an-Average-of-315000-for-Medical-Expenses#:~:text=The%202022%20estimate%20for%20single,men%20and%20%24165%2C000%20for%20women

44 Yang, J., Christophi, C. A., & Farioli, A. (2019, February 15). Association Between Push-up Exercise Capacity and Future Cardiovascular Events Among Active Adult Men. Jama Network. Retrieved November 29, 2022, from https://jamanetwork.com/journals/jamanetworkopen/fullarticle/2724778

45 Alfonsi, W. byS. L. R. byD., Laszlo, W. byS., & Alfonsi, R. byD. (2022, September 26). 8 ways doing planks daily transform your body. Lifehack. Retrieved November 29, 2022, from https://www.lifehack.org/292578/7-things-that-will-happen-when-you-do-planking-exercise-every-day

46 Bentley, D. C., Nguyen, C. H., & Thomas, S. G. (2018, December 12). Resting blood pressure reductions following handgrip exercise training and the impact of age and sex: A systematic review and narrative synthesis. Systematic reviews. Retrieved November 29, 2022, from https://www.ncbi.nlm.nih.gov/pmc/articles/PMC6292032/

47 ScienceDaily. (2012, December 13). Ability to sit and rise from the floor is closely correlated with all-cause mortality risk. ScienceDaily. Retrieved November 29, 2022, from https://www.sciencedaily.com/

releases/2012/12/121213085202.htm#:~:text=2-,Ability%20to%20
sit%20and%20rise%20from%20the%20floor%20is,with%20all%2D-
cause%20mortality%20risk&text=Summary%3A,and%20older%20
men%20and%20women

48 ScienceDaily. (2014, December 18). Ability to balance on one
leg may reflect brain health, stroke risk. ScienceDaily. Retrieved
November 29, 2022, from https://www.sciencedaily.com/releas-
es/2014/12/141218210013.htm#:~:text=Summary%3A,peo-
ple%2C%20a%20study%20has%20shown

49 Gebel, K., Ding, D., & Chey, T. (2015, June). Effect of Moderate to
Vigorous Physical Activity on All-Cause Mortality in Middle-aged
and Older Australians. Jama Network. Retrieved November 29,
2022, from https://jamanetwork.com/journals/jamainternalmedi-
cine/fullarticle/2212268